D0758315

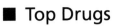 **Top Drugs**

Top Drugs

Their History, Pharmacology, and Syntheses

Jie Jack Li

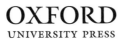

OXFORD
UNIVERSITY PRESS

OXFORD
UNIVERSITY PRESS

Oxford University Press is a department of the
University of Oxford. It furthers the University's objective
of excellence in research, scholarship, and education
by publishing worldwide.

Oxford   New York
Auckland   Cape Town   Dar es Salaam   Hong Kong   Karachi
Kuala Lumpur   Madrid   Melbourne   Mexico City   Nairobi
New Delhi   Shanghai   Taipei   Toronto

With offices in
Argentina   Austria   Brazil   Chile   Czech Republic   France   Greece
Guatemala   Hungary   Italy   Japan   Poland   Portugal   Singapore
South Korea   Switzerland   Thailand   Turkey   Ukraine   Vietnam

Oxford is a registered trade mark of Oxford University Press
in the UK and certain other countries.

Published in the United States of America by
Oxford University Press
198 Madison Avenue, New York, NY 10016

Library of Congress Cataloging-in-Publication Data
Li, Jie Jack.
Top drugs : Their History, Pharmacology, and Syntheses / Jie Jack Li.
pages   cm
Includes bibliographical references and index.
ISBN 978-0-19-936258-5 (hardback)
1. Drugs—History.   2. Drugs—Design.   3. Pharmaceutical chemistry.
I. Title.
RS420.L535   2015
615.1—dc23   2015016478

9 8 7 6 5 4 3 2 1

Printed in the United States of America
on acid-free paper

To Prof. Tami Spector

CONTENTS

■ CNS Drugs

■ Drugs to Treat Infectious Diseases

■ Ulcer Drugs

■ PREFACE

This book originated from a short course that I taught at the University of Pittsburgh. My course on the history, pharmacology, and synthesis of drugs has been warmly received by graduate students and senior undergraduate students majoring in chemistry, biology, pre-med, pharmacy, and related topics. Several professors who teach undergraduate organic chemistry asked me to develop a short textbook that will acclimate undergraduates to the "real world" of chemistry and drug discovery.

This book is geared toward undergraduate institutions interested in offering a short course on this topic. Senior undergraduate students and scientists in both academia and industry will also find it useful to understanding the landscape of current drug discovery and development.

This book covers the history, pharmacology, and synthesis of ten top drugs. Each chapter is divided to the following sections:

1 History
2 Pharmacology
   2.1 Mechanism of Action
   2.2 Structure–Activity Relationship
   2.3 Bioavailability, Metabolism, and Toxicology
3 Synthesis
   3.1 Discovery Route
   3.2 Process Route
4 Concluding Remarks
5 References

I am very much indebted to Prof. Neil K. Garg and Dr. Travis C. McMahon at UCLA for proofreading portions of the final version of the manuscript. Their knowledge and input have tremendously enhanced the quality of this book. Any remaining errors are, of course, solely my own responsibility.

As always, I welcome your critique! Please send your comments to this email address: lijiejackli@gmail.com.

Jie Jack Li
August 2014
San Francisco, California

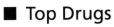

Top Drugs

Cardiovascular Drugs

1   Atorvastatin Calcium (Lipitor)

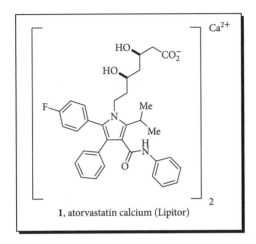

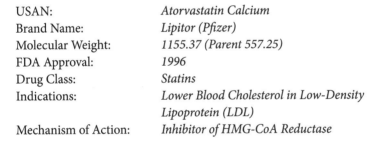

1, atorvastatin calcium (Lipitor)

USAN:	*Atorvastatin Calcium*
Brand Name:	*Lipitor (Pfizer)*
Molecular Weight:	*1155.37 (Parent 557.25)*
FDA Approval:	*1996*
Drug Class:	*Statins*
Indications:	*Lower Blood Cholesterol in Low-Density Lipoprotein (LDL)*
Mechanism of Action:	*Inhibitor of HMG-CoA Reductase*

■ 1 HISTORY

To the human body, cholesterol (**2**) is a Janus-faced molecule. On the one hand, it is an indispensable building block for life—about 23% of total body cholesterol resides in the brain, making up one-tenth of the solid substance of the brain. Red blood cell membranes are also rich in cholesterol, which helps stabilize the cell membranes and protect cells. Furthermore, cholesterol is also the precursor of hormones such as progesterone, testosterone, estrogen, and cortisol. On the other hand, cholesterol helps plaque buildup, which constricts or blocks arteries, leading to angina, heart attack, stroke, and many other cardiovascular diseases. To date, the experimental, genetic, and epidemiologic evidence all point to escalating cholesterol levels as a major risk factor for cardiovascular diseases. Other major risk factors include obesity, diabetes, hypertension, smoking, and inactive lifestyle.

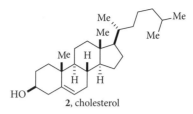

2, cholesterol

Depending on different water-soluble carriers, cholesterol could have starkly opposing effects on the heart. Cholesterol in low-density lipoprotein (LDL), often known as "bad" cholesterol, is the fundamental carrier of blood cholesterol to body cells. It can slowly build up in the walls of the arteries feeding the brain and heart and can form plaques. In contrast, cholesterol in high-density lipoprotein (HDL), frequently dubbed "good" cholesterol, is a carrier that takes cholesterol away from the arteries and brings it to the liver, where it can be removed from circulation by metabolism. The higher the levels of HDL, the better. In general, women have higher levels of HDL, which may explain why women have longer life expectations than men. Their higher levels of estrogen are somehow correlated to higher HDL-cholesterol levels.

Many attempts have been made to lower cholesterol levels. In the 1950s and 1960s, estrogen was tried but was quickly abandoned because it caused feminizing side effects on men. Thyroid hormone also had unacceptable side effects, such as trembling. Resins such as cholestyramine were used as bile acid sequestrants, or bile acid binding resins. The approach was not popular in patients because they were difficult to swallow—literally. One of the early cholesterol-lowering drugs still in use today is nicotinic acid (3), which has been available since 1955.[1] When nicotinic acid is taken in milligram doses, it functions as a vitamin (vitamin B$_3$). When taken in gram doses, nicotinic acid's cholesterol-lowering properties begin to manifest. It works through binding to a G protein-coupled receptor (GPCR) called "nicotinic acid receptor." The nicotinic acid receptors, present not only in adipocytes but also in the spleen, are responsible for lowering LDL-cholesterol levels.[2] The advantage of nicotinic acid is that it also boosts the levels of HDL cholesterol. The disadvantage of nicotinic acid is that it often causes flushing as a side effect.

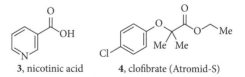

3, nicotinic acid   4, clofibrate (Atromid-S)

In 1954, Imperial Chemical Industries (ICI) discovered that clofibrate (4, Atromid-S) possessed significant cholesterol-lowering activity and marketed it in 1958.[3] Parke-Davis's gemfibrozil (5, Lopid), launched in 1982, was the second fibrate on the market. In order to find safer analogs of clofibrate (4), Parke-Davis screened over 8000 compounds similar to clofibrate using animals. Abbott's fenofibrate (6, Tricor), is also a clofibrate analog. Fibrates have been found to be *peroxisome proliferator-*

activated *receptor-α* (PPARα) agonists. Recent studies have also shown that the risk of drug-drug interactions (DDIs) increases 1,400-fold for statins if they are combined with fibrates. Therefore, fibrates should not be taken with statins.

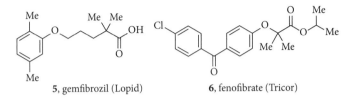

5, gemfibrozil (Lopid)   6, fenofibrate (Tricor)

The best class of cholesterol-lowering drugs are the statins, whose mechanism of action (MOA) is by inhibiting an enzyme in the liver called 3-*hydroxy-3-methyl-glutaryl-CoA* (HMG-CoA, **7**) reductase that promotes the rate-determining step (RDS) in cholesterol biosynthesis cascade. The first statin, mevastatin (Compactin, **8**), was discovered by Akira Endo at Sankyo in Japan in 1973 after screening more than 6000 microbial strains. It is a secondary metabolite of the fungus *Penicillium notatum*. Sankyo conducted a clinical trial with mevastatin (**8**) in 1979 on patients with hypercholesterolemia, but terminated it a year-and-a-half later when intestinal tumors were observed in dogs given mevastatin (**8**) at large doses.

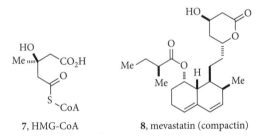

7, HMG-CoA   8, mevastatin (compactin)

Merck was the first to bring a statin to the market in 1987 with their lovastatin (**9**, Mevacor). In 1974, Merck found a potent HMG-CoA reductase inhibitor in the 18th sample that they screened from a collection of soil cultures. The compound from the culture broth of the microorganism *Aspergillus terreus* was lovastatin (**9**). Further efforts to find a drug superior to lovastatin (**9**) were fruitless. Merck carried out semi-total synthesis of lovastatin and arrived at simvastatin (**10**, Zocor), which was 2.5 times more potent than lovastatin (**9**). Zocor's sales peaked in 2003 with annual sales of $5.51 billion.

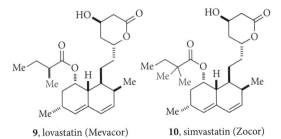

9, lovastatin (Mevacor)   10, simvastatin (Zocor)

In 1991, Bristol-Myers Squibb (BMS) brought Endo/Sankyo's pravastatin (**11**) to the US market with the trade name Pravachol. After dogs were given mevastatin (**8**), Pravachol was isolated from the urine. The dog's liver enzyme CYP450 oxidized mevastatin to Pravachol. The fourth member of the statin class was fluvastatin sodium (**12**, Lescol) by Sandoz (now Novartis). It was the first statin on the market that was a totally synthetic drug. (That is, it was neither a natural product nor a semi-synthesized drug from a natural product.)

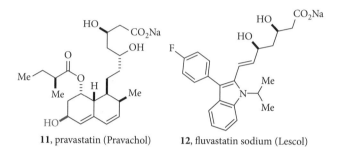

11, pravastatin (Pravachol)   **12**, fluvastatin sodium (Lescol)

Atorvastatin calcium (**1**, Lipitor), the fifth statin to appear on the market, was also prepared by total synthesis. Discovered by scientists at Parke-Davis at the end of the 1980s, it was launched in 1996. It rapidly became the best-selling drug ever, becoming a blockbuster drug in the first year. By the time Lipitor's patent expired at the end of 2011, it had generated over $130 billion in sales for Pfizer, which had acquired Parke-Davis/Warner-Lambert in 2000.

Bayer's cerivastatin (**13**, Baycol) was launched in 1997 but was withdrawn in 2001 largely due to rhabdomyolysis (muscle weakness) stemming from its DDI issues. Cerivastatin is metabolized by CYP3A4, which is the same enzyme used by fibrates such as gemfibrozil (**5**, Lopid) for metabolism. Therefore, they are counterindicated and cannot be taken together. The final statin is AstraZeneca's rosuvastatin (**14**, Crestor), which was introduced in 2003 in the United States. AstraZeneca licensed the drug from Shionogi in Japan.

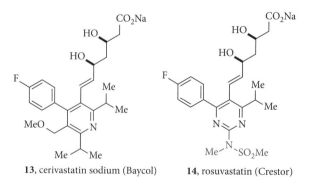

13, cerivastatin sodium (Baycol)   **14**, rosuvastatin (Crestor)

■ 2 PHARMACOLOGY

2.1 Mechanism of Action

Cholesterol in the human body comes from two sources. One is from intestinal absorption of dietary cholesterol. The other source is cholesterol generated inside the body, primarily in the liver, to meet the body's need if the diet is lacking sufficient cholesterol. The liver makes about 70% of the body's cholesterol—three or four times more cholesterol than we get from diet on average. Statins lower cholesterol levels by inhibiting the hepatic HMG-CoA reductase.

In the early 1960s, Bloch elucidated the cholesterol biosynthesis pathway—the process by which the body makes cholesterol. The pathway involves the "acetic acid → squalene → cholesterol" cascade.[4] An early step, which is also the slowest and thus the rate-limiting step, involves the reduction of HMG-CoA to mevalonate, which is then transformed into cholesterol after several additional steps. The crucial reduction process is accomplished by an enzyme called HMG-CoA reductase, which, in turn, is the rate-controlling enzyme in the biosynthetic pathway for cholesterol. Therefore, it is reasonable to believe that if one could block the function of HMG-CoA reductase, the chain reaction for cholesterol production would be suppressed.

HMG-CoA reductase is a polytopic, transmembrane protein that catalyzes a key step in the mevalonate pathway, which is involved in the synthesis of sterols, isoprenoids, and other lipids. Atorvastatin (**1**) binds tightly to the catalytic domain of the HMG-CoA reductase.[5]

2.2 Structure–Activity Relationship

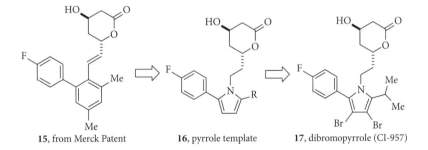

15, from Merck Patent   **16**, pyrrole template   **17**, dibromopyrrole (CI-957)

Inspired by Merck's patent on totally synthetic HMG-CoA reductase inhibitors such as diphenyl **15**,[6–8] medicinal chemists at Parke-Davis (led by Roth) sought to replace the hexahydronaphthalene core with heterocycles.[9,10] Their initial efforts on 1,2,5-tri-substituted pyrroles (**16**) met with disappointment because of low potency. Overlapping pyrroles **16** with Merck's diphenyl **15** quickly revealed that there was un-filled space at the 3- and 4-positions of pyrrole **16**. Dibomopyrrole **17** (CI-957) was thus prepared and it was equipotent to lovastatin (**9**). Unfortunately, dibomopyrrole **17** was tested for use as an extremely potent rodenticide; it

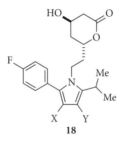

TABLE 1.1. *The Structure-Activity Relationship (SAR) for Atorvastatin*

Entry	X	Y	HMGR Inhibition, IC_{50} (nM)
1	CO_2Et	Ph	50
2	(±)-Ph	CO_2Et	200
3	4-CN-Ph	CO_2Et	280
4	(±)-Ph	CO_2Bn	40
5	(±)-Ph	CONHPh	25 (CI-971)
6	(+)-Ph	CONHPh	7 [(+)-**30**]
7	(−)-Ph	CONHPh	500 [(−)-**30**]

was immediately withdrawn from development due to serious concerns over its toxicities.

Parke-Davis's subsequent endeavor, replacing the 3- and 4-positions of pyrrole **15** with non-halogens, was more fruitful. As shown in Table 1.1, the structure-activity relationship (SAR) is presented as measured by the IC_{50} of the compound's (**18**'s) ability to inhibit the HMG-CoA reductase (HMGR) in the in vitro binding assays. Here, IC_{50} is the concentration of the compound that showed half maximal inhibitory effect to the HMG-CoA reductase enzyme.

For entry 1, pyrrole **18** is substituted with an ethyl ester at the 3-position and a phenyl group at the 4-position. It was half as potent as lovastatin (**9**, IC_{50} ~23 nM). Compounds in entries 2 and 3 are not potent enough. Entry 4 shows a pyrrole substituted with a phenyl group at the 3-position and a benzyl ester at the 4-position. It was getting close to the potency of lovastatin (**9**). However, esters as drugs are often not bioavailable—esterase can easily hydrolyze the esters to their corresponding carboxylic acids. One of the most frequently used bioisosteres for an ester is an amide. Entry 5 showed a pyrrole where the benzyl ester at the 4-position was replaced with a phenyl amide, which is almost equipotent to lovastatin (**9**). The compound was designated as CI-971.

However, CI-971 is a racemate, consisting of two enantiomers. Separation of those two enantiomers resulted in a compound with a positive rotation and one with a negative. The one with a positive rotation (+)-**30** (Entry 6) has an IC_{50} of 7 nM in vitro and was designated as CI-981, which would in time become atorvastatin calcium and Lipitor. It is remarkable that the enantiomer of CI-981 [(−)-**30**] in entry 7 is 71-fold less potent!

2.3 Bioavailability, Metabolism, and Toxicology

Drug metabolism is a defense mechanism to remove foreign compounds or xenobiotics that have made their way into the body. Metabolism is considered a detoxification pathway by which the molecules are chemically modified to make them more polar, thereby facilitating elimination from the body and rendering them pharmacologically inactive. Avoiding unwanted toxicity is always desirable in all situations, and although active metabolites are generally unwanted they can sometimes provide additional pharmacological activity in certain situations that may be beneficial—for example, a metabolite which is formed at the site of action or an active metabolite formed from a rapidly metabolized parent drug (e.g., prodrug). Atorvastatin (**1**, Lipitor) is such an example. It is metabolized by cytochrome P450 3A4 (CYP3A4) in the liver to two aromatic hydroxylated metabolites (**19** and **20**, respectively): both metabolites are pharmacologically active and formed in the liver, which is the target organ for lowering cholesterol.[11-13] Among the statins, atorvastatin, along with lovastatin (**9**) and simvastatin (**10**), are metabolized by CYP3A4, while fluvastatin (**12**) is metabolized by CYP2C9. Cerivastatin (**13**) is subject to two metabolic pathways mediated by CYP2C8 and 3A4, whereas pravastatin (**11**) and rosuvastatin (**14**) undergo little metabolism.[14,15]

The fact that cerivastatin (**13**) is mainly metabolized by CYP2C8 and 3A4 is the root of its drug-drug interaction (DDI). As mentioned before, since fibrates such as gemfibrozil (**5**, Lopid) are also metabolized by CYP3A4, rhabdomyolysis (muscle weakness) ensued when cerivastatin (**13**) and gemfibrozil (**5**) were given together.

Atorvastatin (**1**) has high solubility and high permeability. As a consequence, it has complete intestinal absorption. However, the drug is probably subjected to first-pass metabolism by oxidation and glucuronidation in the gut wall and the liver. After oral administration, bioavailability (F%) is 14%. As mentioned earlier, CYP3A4 is responsible for the formation of two active oxidative metabolites from the acid and lactone forms of atorvastatin in vivo; the drug is completely metabolized in vivo; and the metabolites **19** and **20** are eliminated by biliary secretion and direct secretion from blood to intestine. The total plasma clearance of atorvastatin acid is 625 mL/min and the elimination half-life is ~7 h. The renal route is of minor importance (<1%) for the elimination of atorvastatin acid and its metabolites and renal failure does not affect their elimination.[16]

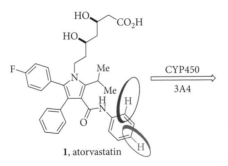

1, atorvastatin

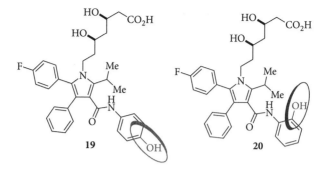

As far as toxicology is concerned, atorvastatin (**1**) is the gold standard in terms of safety as well as efficacy for statins. Extensive data from randomized clinical trials, post-marketing analyses, and reports to regulatory agencies demonstrated the safety of atorvastatin (**1**) in a large number of patients with a variety of indications. With the exception of a slightly higher rate of liver enzyme elevations with atorvastatin (**1**) at the highest dosage that the FDA approved (80 mg/day), which does not appear to confer an increased risk of clinically important adverse events, atorvastatin (**1**) is notable for its lack of dose-dependent tolerability. Unlike simvastatin (**10**), atorvastatin (**1**) is associated with a low incidence of muscular toxicity at all therapeutic dosages. It is not associated with adverse neurological or cognitive effects, and has a placebo-like effect on the kidney as a result of its favorable pharmacokinetic profile, which is unique among the statins. Atorvastatin (**1**) is generally well-tolerated in elderly patients, with no dose-dependent increase in adverse events up to the maximum daily dosage of 80 mg/day. Thus, atorvastatin (**1**) is a safe and well-tolerated agent for use in patients requiring lipid-lowering therapy.[17]

■ 3 SYNTHESIS

3.1 Discovery Route

The first synthesis of atorvastatin (**1**) was a small-scale synthesis by Parke-Davis discovery chemistry using a racemic synthesis followed by separation of diastereomers.[9,10] Although several methods had been used previously to synthesize the central pyrrole ring of related, less highly substituted pyrrole HMGR inhibitors in discovery chemistry, synthesis of the penta-substituted pyrrole ring of atorvastatin was first accomplished by the [3 + 2]-cycloaddition reaction of an acetylenic amide with an α-amido acid.

Thus, as shown in Scheme 2 alkylation of the ethylene glycol acetal of 3-amino-1-propanal (**22**) with α-bromoester **21** afforded an α-amino acid ester (**23**) that after formation of the amide with isobutyryl chloride and hydrolysis provided the α-amido acid substrate (**24**) required for the [3 + 2]-cycloaddition reaction. Heating **24** in acetic anhydride in the presence of excess 3-phenyl-propynoic acid phenylamide (**25**) afforded the [3 + 2]-cycloaddition adduct **26**, presumably through addition of the acetylene to the oxazolone intermediate derived from **24**, followed by extrusion of CO_2. As in similar [3 + 2]-cycloadditions, the reaction was highly regioselective, forming essentially only one of the two possible regioisomeric products (**26**).

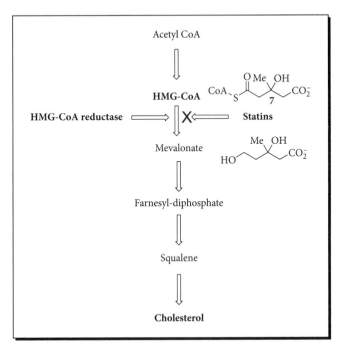

Scheme 1. The Mevalonate Pathway: The Role of HMG-CoA Reductase and Statins in the Production of Cholesterol

The masked aldehyde in **26** was most efficiently unveiled in a two-step, one-pot procedure by first converting **26** to the diethyl acetal, followed by acid hydrolysis to aldehyde **27**. Reaction of **27** with the dianion of methyl acetoacetate introduced (±)-**28** with all of the carbons required for the mevalonolactone as well as the 5-hydroxyl, although this center was introduced in a racemic fashion. Application of the diastereoselective reduction procedure employing n-Bu$_3$B and NaBH$_4$ at low temperature (−78 °C) produced the 3,5-diol as a 9:1 mixture of the desired *syn*-diol (±)-**29** to the undesired *anti*-diol. Hydrolysis of the ester followed by lactonization in refluxing toluene produced the racemic lactone of atorvastatin as a 9:1 mixture of *trans/cis* diastereoisomers (±)-**30** in an overall yield of 66% from (±)-**28**. One recrystallization of (±)-**30** raised this ratio to >97:3 *trans/cis*.

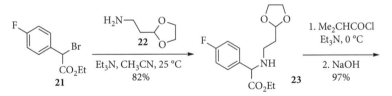

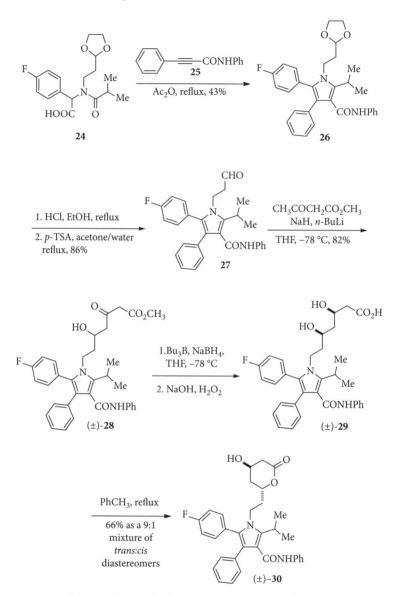

Scheme 2. Racemic Synthesis of Atorvastatin Lactone [(±)–30]

The interesting mechanism for which **26** was prepared via the [3 + 2]-cycloaddition from amidyl-acid **24** and alkyne **25** warrants further explanations. In refluxing acetic anhydride, amidyl-acid **24** forms mixed anhydride **31**, which cyclizes to provide intermediate **32** (Scheme 2). Deprotonation of **32** then affords 1,3-dipole **33** (a *meso-ionic* heterocycle, an isomer of the oxazolone intermediate), which undergoes the [3 + 2]-cycloaddition with alkyne **25** to form adduct **34**. Subsequent CO_2 extrusion then affords pyrrole **26**.

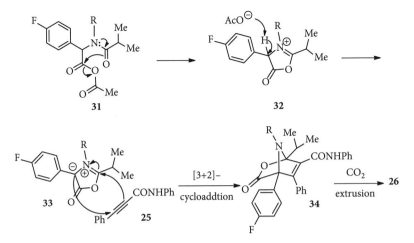

Scheme 3. The Mechanism of the [3 + 2]-Cycloaddition to Form Adduct **26**

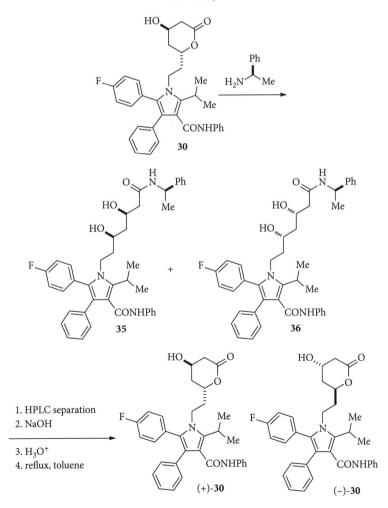

Scheme 4. Separation of Enantiomers

With racemic atorvastatin lactone (**30**) in hand, separation of the two enantiomers was accomplished by preparation of the diastereomeric (R)-α-methylbenzyl amides **35** and **36**, separation by HPLC, and hydrolysis and re-lactonization to produce 94% optically pure (+)-**30** (Scheme 3), a procedure used effectively to separate an analogous pair of HMG-CoA reductase (HMGR) inhibitors by Lynch et al.[18]

3.2 Process Route

With so much money at stake, numerous process routes have been developed all over the world.[19-21] The original process route developed by Parke-Davis's Process Chemistry is shown in Scheme 5. This highly convergent approach takes advantage of the Paal-Knorr synthesis of penta-substituted pyrroles from the fully substituted diketone **37** and the fully functionalized, stereochemically pure side-chain **38**. Thus, under very carefully defined conditions (1 equiv. pivalic acid, 1:4:1 toluene-heptane-THF, a process optimized in one whole year!) pyrrole **39** was constructed in 75% yield. Deprotection and formation of the hemi-calcium salt produced stereochemically pure atorvastatin calcium (**1**) in a convergent, high-yielding and commercially viable manner.[19,20]

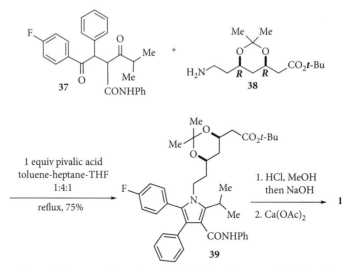

Scheme 5. Convergent, Enantiospecific Synthesis of Atorvastatin Calcium (**1**)

On the other hand, diketone **37** was prepared by taking advantage of the Stetter reaction (Scheme 6). Thus, condensation of commercially available isobutyrylacetanilide **40** with benzaldehyde in the presence of β-alanine and acetic acid afforded the enone **41** in 85% yield. Treatment of this enone with 4-fluorobenzaldehyde under the Stetter conditions, utilizing N-ethylthiazolium catalyst **42** under anhydrous conditions produced the highly substituted 1,4-diketone **37** in 80% yield.[21]

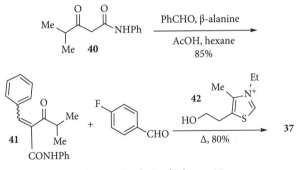

Scheme 6. Synthesis of Diketone **37**

Meanwhile, the fully decorated amine **38** was assembled from the commercially available alcohol–ester **43**, a compound which has also been the subject of considerable process development due to its use as a common intermediate in the synthesis of several other HMGR inhibitors. Conversion of **43** to the 4-halo- or 4-nitrobenzenesulfonate **44** followed by displacement with sodium cyanide provided the *t*-butyl-ester **45** in 90% yield. It was noted that this procedure was most scalable employing the 4-chlorobenzenesulfonate **44a** due to the instability of the 4-bromo and 4-nitro analogs to aqueous hydrolysis. Raney-Ni reduction as before provided the fully elaborated side-chain as the *t*-butyl ester **38** (Scheme 7).

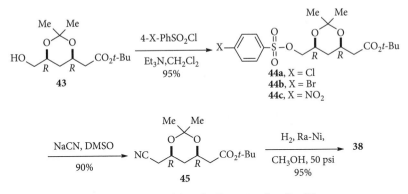

Scheme 7. Synthesis of the Side-Chain **38** as the *t*-Butyl Ester

■ 4 CONCLUDING REMARKS

Atorvastatin calcium (**1**) is the best in class for statins. Its peak sales were $13 billion in 2006. Statins set a high standard in efficacy, a high standard in safety, and a high standard in financial benefits.[22] The discovery of statins marked the golden age of the pharmaceutical industry.

As far as the field of cholesterol reduction is concerned, cholesterol-ester transfer protein (CETP) inhibitors are the next possibilities. CETP is an enzyme in the blood that shuttles cholesterol and triglyceride between LDL and HDL. It was observed that a subpopulation in Japan with CETP deficiency had plasma HDL levels 5–10 times higher than the average population. It was then believed that inhibiting the CETP would boost the HDL levels. The first CETP inhibitor, Pfizer's torcetrapib (**46**), showed efficacy in one of the largest phase III trials (involving 15,000 patients). Unfortunately, those trials were terminated at the end of 2006 when a higher death rate was observed for patients taking torcetrapib with Lipitor than for patients taking Lipitor alone. The known hypertension side effect was the possible cause of the safety issue.[22]

Roche's dalcetrapib (**47**) entered the graveyard of CETP inhibitors in 2012 due to a lack of clinically meaningful efficacy. However, Merck's anatrapib (**48**) is undergoing phase III trials at the time of writing this book. I am eager to learn how it will fare in terms of risk/benefit profile.

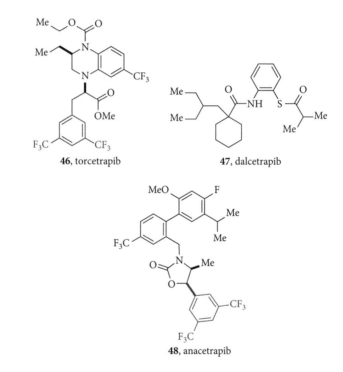

46, torcetrapib   **47**, dalcetrapib

48, anacetrapib

■ 5 REFERENCES

1. Altschul, R.; Hoffer, A.; Stephen, J. D. *Arch Biochem Biophys* **1955**, *54*, 558–559.

2. Karpe, F.; Frayn, K. N. *Lancet* **2004**, *363*, 1892–1894.

3. Thorp, J. M.; Waring, W. S. *Nature* **1962**, *194*, 948–949.

4. Steinberg, D. *J. Lipid Res.* **2005**, *46*, 2037–2051.

5. Istvan, E. S.; Deisenhofer, J. *Science* **2001**, *292*, 1160–1164.

6. Willard, A. K.; Novello, F. C.; Hoffmann, W. F.; Cragoe, E. J., Jr. *(+)-(4R,6S)-(E)-6-[2-(4'-Fluoro-3,3',5-trimethyl-[1,1'-biphenyl]-2-yl)ethenyl]-3,4,5,6-tetrahydro-4-hydroxy-2H-pyran-2-one and a pharmaceutical composition containing it.* Eur. Pat. Appl. (1983), 27 pp.

7. Willard, A. K.; Novello, F. C.; Hoffman, W. F.; Cragoe, Edward J., Jr. *Substituted Pyranone Inhibitors of Cholesterol Synthesis*. USP 4,567,289 (1986). 24 pp. Cont.-in-part of U.S. 4,459,423.

8. Stokker, G. E.; Alberts, A. W.; Anderson, P. S. et al. *J. Med. Chem*. 1986, *29*, 170–181.

9. Roth, B. D.; Ortwine, D. F.; Hoefle, M. L.; Stratton, C. D.; Sliskovic, D. R.; Wilson, M. W.; Newton, R. S. *J. Med. Chem*. **1990**, *33*, 21–31.

10. Roth, B. D.; Blankley, C. J.; Chucholowski, A. W. et al. *J. Med. Chem*. **1991**, *34*, 357–366.

11. Black, A. E.; Sinz, M. W.; Hayes, R. N.; Woolf, T. F. *Drug Metab. Dispos*. **1998**, *26*, 755–763.

12. Jacobsen, W.; Kuhn, B.; Soldner, A.; Kirchner, G.; Sewing, K.-F.; Kollman, P. A.; Benet, L. Z.; Christians, U. *Drug Metab. Dispos*. **2000**, *28*, 1369–1378.

13. Park, J.-E.; Kim, K.-B.; Bae, S. K.; Moon, B.-S.; Liu, K.-H.; Shin, J.-G. *Xenobiotica* **2008**, *38*, 1240–1251.

14. Christians, U.; Jacobsen, W.; Floren, L. C. *Pharmacol. Ther*. **1998**, *80*, 1–34.

15. Shitara, Y.; Sugiyama, Y. *Pharmacol. Ther*. **2006**, *112*, 71–105.

16. Lennernas, H. *Clin. Pharmacokinet*. **2003**, *42*, 1141–1160.

17. Arca, M. *Drugs* **2007**, *67(Suppl. 1)*, 63–69.

18. Lynch, J. E.; Volante, R. P.; Wattley, R. V.; Shinkai, I. *Tetrahedron Lett*. **1987**, *28*, 1385–1388.

19. Baumann, K. L.; Butler, D. E.; Deering, C. F.; Mennen, K. E.; Millar, A.; Nanninga, T. N.; Palmer, C. W.; Roth, B. D. *Tetrahedron Lett*. **1992**, *33*, 2283–2284.

20. Wade, R. A.; Zennie, T. M.; Briggs, C. A.; Jennings, R. A.; Nanninga, T. N.; Palmer, C. W.; Clay, R. J. *Org. Process Res. Develop*. **1997**, *1*, 320–324.

21. Browner, P. L.; Butler, D. E.; Deering, C. F.; Le, T. V.; Millar, A.; Nanninga, T. N.; Roth, B. D. *Tetrahedron Lett*. **1992**, *33*, 2279–2282.

22. Li, J. J. *Triumph of the Heart—The Story of Statins*, Oxford University Press: New York, 2009.

2 Clopidogrel Bisulfate (Plavix)

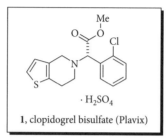

1, clopidogrel bisulfate (Plavix)

USAN:	*Clopidogrel Bisulfate*
Brand Name:	*Plavix (Sanofi-Aventis/Bristol-Myers Squibb)*
Molecular Weight:	*419.90 (Parent 321.06)*
FDA Approval:	*1993*
Drug Class:	*Anti-Platelet*
Indications:	*Antithrombotic, Blood Thinner*
Mechanism of Action:	*Antagonist of the P2Y$_{12}$ Purinergic Receptor*

■ 1 HISTORY

Three types of blood cells exist in the human body: red blood cells, white blood cells, and platelets. Red blood cells, 45% of the blood, transport oxygen from the lungs to other body parts. White cells, less than 1% of the blood, defend us against bacterial and viral invasions. Platelets, also less than 1% of the blood (55% of the remaining blood is plasma), are small cell fragments that are involved in helping the blood clot, a process known as blood coagulation. Coagulation takes place when the enzyme thrombin elicits platelets and fibrin, a blood protein. Without platelets, coagulation at the site of an injury does not occur and uncontrolled bleeding ensues. Individuals with no ability to clot have a genetic condition called hemophilia. These individuals must periodically administer a clotting factor to their blood to prevent constant bleeding.

Conversely, thrombosis, the formation of blood clots *inside* blood vessels, can block coronary arteries and constrict vital oxygen supplies, resulting in a heart attack or stroke. Coronary thrombosis is a life-threatening blood clot in the artery. Deep-vein thrombosis (DVT) is commonly associated with long-distance air travel, when passengers are confined to cramped spaces for many hours.

In contrast with thrombosis, in which the clot is stationary, embolus is when an object such as a clot migrates from one part of the body through blood circulation and causes blockage. A pulmonary embolism occurs when emboli travel to the lungs. Approximately 90% of heart attacks and 80% of strokes are caused by blood clots, which kill some 200,000 hospital patients in the US each year.

Anticoagulants (blood thinners) are the drugs of choice to prevent and treat both thrombosis and embolism. To date, heparin, warfarin, and aspirin have all been widely used as blood thinners to prevent blood clots from forming.

Heparin is one of the oldest medicines still in widespread clinical use. Heparin was extracted in 1916 by Jay McLean from dog's liver in the laboratories of William Howell at the Johns Hopkins University.[1] Nearly a century after its discovery, heparin is still extensively used in clinics during hemodialysis, vascular surgery, and organ transplantation. Large dose heparin injections are routinely used to prevent blood clots in patients undergoing kidney dialysis or heart surgery. Heparin is also used to coat stents, flexible mesh metal cylinders that act as scaffolding to prevent an artery from collapsing after an obstruction has been cleared in a procedure called angioplasty, eliminating the need for a patient to take anti-clotting drugs. Heparin prevents formation of blood clots that block the artery at the site of the cleared obstruction.

Heparin works by binding to the active sites on the surface of the plasma protein antithrombin, converting this "sleeping" serine protease inhibitor antithrombin III (also known as AT III) to a potent anticoagulant.

Protamine sulfate has been used as an antidote in cases of heparin overdose to reverse heparin's anticoagulant effects by binding to it.

Today, there are three types of heparins in use:

A. Natural heparins, known as unfractionated heparins, have a long range of molecular weights (from 3,000 to 15,000). The larger the molecular weight the longer the heparin stays in the body; there is always a risk of bleeding when large heparins stay in the body longer than necessary.

B. Small molecular-weight heparins are fragments of natural heparins produced by controlled enzymatic or chemical depolymerization processes that yield polysaccharide chains with a mean molecular weight of about 5,000.

C. Pentasaccharides are synthetic drugs that only contain the five key sugar units. The first commercial sulfated pentasaccharide, fondaparinux (**2**), has been on the market since 2001. With a half-life of 17 hours, fondaparinux (**2**) has to be given once daily by subcutaneous administration. The other pentasaccharide, *idraparinux* (**3**), the hypermethylated fondaparinux, with a half-life of 80 hours, is the longest-acting pentasaccharide, and only needs to be given once a week.[2]

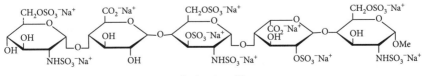

fondaparinux (**2**)

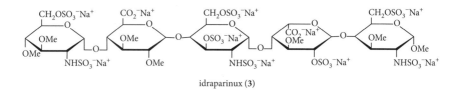

idraparinux (3)

While heparins have to be given intravenously (it decomposes in the gut), Warfarin (**5**), available since the early 1950s, is an oral anticoagulant. In 1939, Karl Paul Link at the University of Wisconsin–Madison isolated dicumarol (**4**) from spoiled sweet clover hay that killed many cows. Cumarol (**4**) was produced when the sweet clovers were oxidized during fermentation. Warfarin (**5**, Coumadin), a synthetic analog of dicumarol, is more potent than dicumarol. It also has both higher water solubility and greater bioavailability than dicumarol. Furthermore, warfarin (**5**) and other coumarin analogs have an antidote—vitamin K, which is a key player in the blood clotting cascade. Warfarin's mechanism of action (MOA), in turn, is via inhibition of the vitamin K epoxide reductase as a vitamin K antagonist.[3–5]

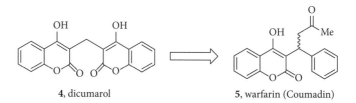

4, dicumarol   5, warfarin (Coumadin)

Warfarin (**5**) is still one of the most prescribed oral anticoagulants. However, it is associated with skin necrosis and hair loss. Moreover, gauging the dosage of warfarin not only depends on factors such as a patient's age and weight, but also on factors such as genetic polymorphism in the genes encoding CYP2C9, the main enzyme responsible for the metabolism of the S-warfarin (the more potent of the two enantiomers), as well as the level of vitamin K epoxide reductase complex, subunit 1 (VKORC1).[6] Even a slight change in dosage can mean the difference between too little, which would not be effective in preventing blood clots, and too much, which can cause dangerous internal bleeding. There is a dire need for more optimal oral anticoagulants.

Aspirin's antiplatelet effect was first discovered by Harvey J. Weiss at Columbia University in 1967.[7] Spurred by Armand Quick's report that low-dose aspirin prolonged the prothrombin (clotting) time in normal subjects, Weiss gave 300-mg aspirin to ten healthy men and observed that aspirin indeed inhibited platelet aggregation and adenosine diphosphate (ADP) release. Meanwhile, many researchers reported that anti-inflammatory agents, including aspirin, inhibited aggregation of platelets in several animal species. Weiss proposed in his *Lancet* paper "the results suggest that these agents may have antithrombotic properties."[7]

Despite aspirin's popularity in treating almost every ill known to man (the world consumes 50 million pounds of aspirin a year); its MOA was not deciphered until 1971. It was found that aspirin works by inhibiting prostaglandin synthetase, explaining most of its antiplatelet, antipyretic, and anti-inflammatory properties.[8] Thromboxane A_2 (**6**, TxA_2, Fig. 2.1), a prostaglandin, is known to promote clotting, and low-dose aspirin (81 mg baby aspirin) is currently used as a prophylaxis to decrease the risk of heart attack and occlusive stroke by inhibiting the biosynthesis of thromboxane A_2.

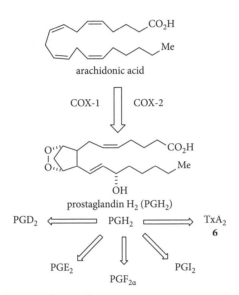

Fig. 2.1. The Arachidonic Acid Cascade

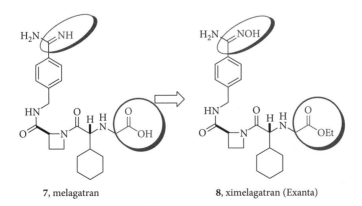

7, melagatran   8, ximelagatran (Exanta)

AstraZeneca's oral anticoagulant ximelagatran (**8**, Exanta), a direct thrombin inhibitor, became available in Europe in the early 2000s. Guided by the three-dimensional coordinates of human α-thrombin, medicinal chemists arrived at a dipeptide, melagatran (**7**). Unfortunately, melagatran is highly ionic, with an oral bioavailability of less than 3–7% in humans although its bioavailability was greater than 50% in dogs. Transforming the original carboxylic acid to in the corresponding ethyl ester and converting the original amidine, a strong base, to hydroxyamidine, a nearly neutral fragment, gave rise to ximelagatran (**8**). In essence, ximelagatran is a double pro-drug of melagatran (**7**) with an oral bioavailability of 18–20% in humans.[9]

One disadvantage of ximelagatran (**8**) is that there is no antidote if acute bleeding develops whereas warfarin (**5**) can be antagonized by vitamin K and heparins by protamine sulfate. Another drawback of ximelagatran (**8**) is its effect of severe liver toxicity in a small population of patients; this was one of the reasons why in 2004 the FDA rejected the drug for licensure in the US. In 2006, AstraZeneca withdrew ximelagatran (**8**) from the market after additional reports of liver damage surfaced.[10]

The brightest star in the universe of anticoagulants is Sanofi-Aventis's clopidogrel bisulfate (**1**, Plavix), which was an improvement on one of their earlier drugs: ticlopidine hydrochloride (**10**, Ticlid).

In 1972, Maffrand of Porcor (later Sanofi) prepared some analogs of tinoridine (**9**, Nonflamin), a thienopyridine antiinflammatory drug discovered by the Japanese drug firm Yoshitomi. Maffrand's thienopyridine analogs were not endowed with antiinflammatory properties at all; instead, they inhibited blood platelet aggregation. Maffrand's group prepared and evaluated hundreds of similar compounds to determine which produced optimum antiplatelet aggregation. The fruit of their 5-year labor was Ticlid (**10**), whose marketing was approved in France in 1978.[11]

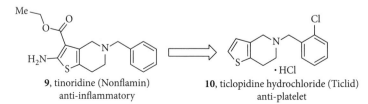

9, tinoridine (Nonflamin)
anti-inflammatory

10, ticlopidine hydrochloride (Ticlid)
anti-platelet

Unfortunately, thrombotic thrombocytopenic purpura (TTP), a rare but potentially fatal side effect, was observed in patients after Ticlid (**10**) reached the market.[12] Because of TTP and other side effects, when Ticlid was approved by the FDA in 1991 the agency required it to carry a "black box" warning that it could cause life-threatening blood disorders. As a consequence, the sales of Ticlid were insignificant.

Efforts at Sanofi to seek a safer drug with equal or higher potency by minimizing Ticlid's toxicities resulted in clopidogrel bisulfate (**1**, Plavix). Clopidogrel bisulfate (**1**) provides a significant improvement in the prevention of myocardial infarction, stroke and vascular death in patients with symptomatic atherosclerosis (ischemic stroke, myocardial infarction, or established peripheral arterial disease).[13]

In 1997, the FDA granted clearance to market Plavix (**1**) for the reduction of atherosclerotic events (myocardial infarction, stroke, vascular deaths) in patients with atherosclerosis documented by recent myocardial infarctions, recent stroke, or established peripheral arterial diseases. The drug also won approval by the European Commission in 1998. It quickly became widely used in angioplasty procedures to open clogged arteries in the heart and legs and to prevent strokes. Within the first year, more than three million patients in America had taken Plavix, partially because of its improved clinical outcomes and safety benefits in patients with acute coronary syndrome (ACS). More than 48 million Americans use Plavix on a daily basis.[14,15] Plavix was the second best-selling drugs of all time from 2008 to 2011.

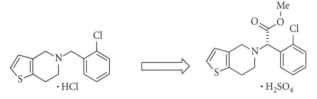

10, ticlopidine hydrochloride (Ticlid)   **1**, clopidogrel bisulfate (Plavix)

■ 2 PHARMACOLOGY

2.1 Bioavailability, Metabolism, and Toxicology

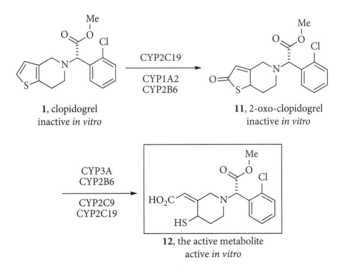

1, clopidogrel
inactive *in vitro*

11, 2-oxo-clopidogrel
inactive *in vitro*

12, the active metabolite
active *in vitro*

Scheme 1. *In vivo* Metabolism of Clopidogrel (**1**)

Remarkably, despite clopidogrel's (**1**) enormous commercial success, the identity of its active metabolite **12** was not known until 1999, when it was isolated after exposure of clopidogrel (**1**) or 2-oxo-clopidogrel (**11**) to human hepatic microsomes

(Scheme 1).[16] Metabolite **12** was determined to be an antagonist of the $P2Y_{12}$ purinergic receptor; it prevents binding of ADP to the $P2Y_{12}$ receptor. However, clopidogrel (**1**) itself is not active in vitro, but is activated in vivo by cytochrome P450 (CYP450)-mediated hepatic metabolism to give the active metabolite **12**.[17]

As far as the pharmacokinetics (PK) of clopidogrel (**1**) is concerned, clopidogrel is rapidly absorbed with a T_{max} reached at from 0.5 to 1.0 h.[18] Because clopidogrel (**1**) is a prodrug, it takes 37 days for its effect on platelet aggregation to reach the steady state. Therefore, a common regimen entails a 300-mg loading dose (LD), followed by 75-mg maintenance dose (MD). Generally, C_{max} for the active metabolite **12** is 70 ng/mL and 28 ng/mL for a 300-mg LD and a 75-mg MD, respectively. The corresponding area under the curve (AUC_{0-t}) is 90 ng•h/mL and 29 ng•h/mL, respectively, for a 300-mg/75-mg LD/MD regimen. The concentrations of active metabolite **12** are typically below the assay limit (0.5 ng/mL) 2 to 4 h after dosing, therefore its half-life $T_{1/2}$ could not be calculated.

Similarly, ticlopidine (**10**) is first oxidized by CYP450 in the liver to 2-oxo-ticlopidine (**13**), which is further oxidized to the active metabolite **14**.[18] Just like metabolite **12**, metabolite **14** was also determined to be an antagonist of the $P2Y_{12}$ purinergic receptor and prevents binding of ADP to the $P2Y_{12}$ receptor. Note that clopidogrel (**1**) and ticlopidine (**10**) do *not* share a common active metabolite although both active metabolites **12** and **14** are $P2Y_{12}$ receptor antagonists (Scheme 2).

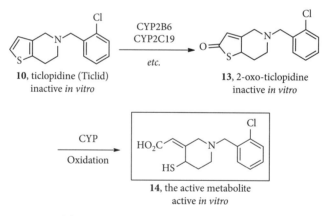

10, ticlopidine (Ticlid)
inactive *in vitro*

13, 2-oxo-ticlopidine
inactive *in vitro*

14, the active metabolite
active *in vitro*

Scheme 2. *In vivo* Metabolism of Ticlopidine (**10**)

Ticlopidine (**10**) was plagued by toxicity issues. In addition to TTP, it is known to induce severe bone marrow aplasia, cholestatic jaundice, and acute cholestatic hepatitis. In contrast, clopidogrel (**1**) is associated with fewer toxicity issues. Since CYP450 2C19 (CYP2C19) is involved in metabolizing clopidogrel (**1**) to its active metabolite **12**, patients with certain genetic variations in the CYP2C19 gene may not benefit from taking clopidogrel (**1**). In addition, because proton pump inhibitors (see chap, 10) and antiepileptic drugs are often metabolized by CYP2C19, DDI occur when taken together with clopidogrel (**1**).[19]

2.2 Mechanism of Action

Platelets play an important role in thrombus formation by adhering to exposed subendothelial structures in response to vascular injury. In this way, they become rapidly activated by their interaction with thrombogenic substrates and generated or locally released agonists, including adenosine-5′-diphosphate (ADP), thromboxane A_2 (**6**), and thrombin. On the other hand, ADP plays a key role in hemostasis as well as in the pathogenesis of arterial thrombosis because the pharmacological inhibition of ADP-induced platelet aggregation decreases the risk of arterial thrombosis. The transduction of the ADP signal involves its interaction with two platelet receptors, the G_q-coupled $P2Y_1$ receptor and the G_i-coupled $P2Y_{12}$ receptor, which belong to the family of purinergic P2 receptors. The concomitant activation of both the G_q and G_i pathways by ADP is necessary to elicit normal platelet aggregation (Fig. 2.2). In contrast to $P2Y_1$, $P2Y_{12}$ has a very selective tissue distribution, making it an attractive molecular target for therapeutic intervention. Indeed, metabolites **12** and **14** of thienopyridines ticlopidine (**10**) and clopidogrel (**1**) are both $P2Y_{12}$ antagonists and they are shown to be efficacious antithrombotic agents in clinical practice either alone or in combination with other antithrombotic drugs.[20]

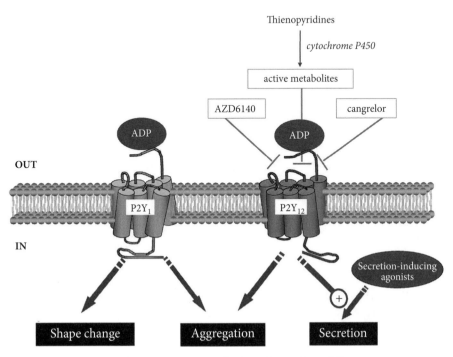

Fig. 2.2. ADP, $P2Y_1$ and $P2Y_{12}$ Receptors in the Coagulation Cascade[20]

2.3 Structure–Activity Relationship

The contemporary sense of SAR for clopidogrel (**1**) does not exist because it is a prodrug and is not active in vitro as an antagonist for the $P2Y_{12}$ purinergic receptor. On the contrary, the SAR was carried out using in vivo animal testing. While this was the common modus operandi 50 years ago, modern drug discovery mostly takes advantage of the rational drug design, exploring the inhibitory ability or the antagonism of the drug to either the enzyme or the receptor. But occasionally, the old-fashioned animal models still get the job done. In addition to clopidogrel (**1**), ezetimibe (Zetia) is another recent example of carrying out the SAR investigations using animal models.[21]

In light of ticlopidine's (**10**) shortcomings, a safer drug with equal or higher potency was desired. Back in 1975, Sanofi synthesized a ticlopidine derivative by adding a methyl group at the bridging carbon to give the "(±)-methyl-ticlopidine (±)-**15**." The "right-handed" isomer (+)-**15** was inactive; and the "left-handed" isomer (−)-**15** was active but was still more toxic than ticlopidine (**10**).[22] Needless to say, the development of the "methyl-ticlopidine" was not continued.

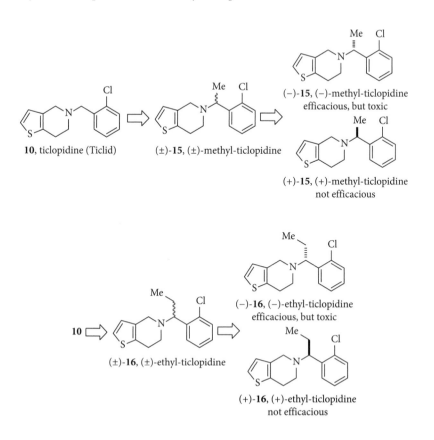

10, ticlopidine (Ticlid)

(±)-**15**, (±)-methyl-ticlopidine

(−)-**15**, (−)-methyl-ticlopidine
efficacious, but toxic

(+)-**15**, (+)-methyl-ticlopidine
not efficacious

(±)-**16**, (±)-ethyl-ticlopidine

(−)-**16**, (−)-ethyl-ticlopidine
efficacious, but toxic

(+)-**16**, (+)-ethyl-ticlopidine
not efficacious

Similarly, the "ethyl-ticlopidine (±)-**16**" was also prepared in 1978. It was even more toxic than ticlopidine (**10**). To make matters worse, both isomers (–)-**16** and (+)-**16** were less potent than ticlopidine (**10**). Not surprisingly, they were subsequently abandoned as well.

In July 1980, Sanofi prepared the methyl ester [(±)-**1**] substituted on the bridge carbon of the ticlopidine molecule. The corresponding HCl salt was prepared and designated as PCR 4099; it was both more potent and better tolerated than ticlopidine (**10**). Regrettably, PCR 4099 [(±)-**1**] caused convulsions in rats, mice, and baboons at certain high dosages. To determine whether each enantiomer behaved differently in terms of potency and toxicity, the enantiomers of the racemate PCR 4099 [(±)-**1**] were separated. The "left-handed" isomer (–)-**1** had no significant platelet inhibition activity; but the "right-handed" isomer (+)-1 was potent and better tolerated than ticlopidine (**10**). More gratifyingly, the "right-handed" isomer (+)-**1** did not cause convulsion in animals at dosages that both PCR 4099 [(±)-**1**] and the "left-handed" isomer [(–)-**1**] did. Moreover, the inactive (–)-(**1**) isomer is 40 times less well-tolerated than its corresponding (+)-enantiomer. Therefore, it is clearly advantageous to choose (+)-clopidogrel [(+)-**1**] as the drug candidate.

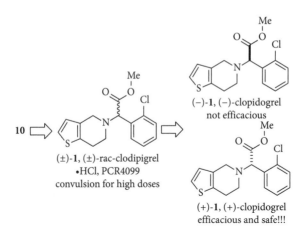

(±)-**1**, (±)-rac-clodipigrel
•HCl, PCR4099
convulsion for high doses

(–)-**1**, (–)-clopidogrel
not efficacious

(+)-**1**, (+)-clopidogrel
efficacious and safe!!!

■ 3 SYNTHESIS

3.1 Discovery Route

The original Sanofi synthesis of (±)-clopidogrel [(±)-**1**] began with the formation of the methyl ester **18** (Scheme 3), which was prepared using the Fischer esterification by refluxing chlorinated mandelic acid **17** with methanol in the presence of concentrated HCl.[23] Chlorination of **18** using thionyl chloride gave methyl α-chloro-(2-chlorophenyl)acetate (**19**). Subsequent S_N2 displacement of 19 with thieno[3,2-*c*]pyridine (**20**) then delivered (±)-clopidogrel [(±)-**1**].

Alternatively, α-bromo-(2-chlorophenyl)acetic acid (**21**) was prepared by treatment of 2-chlorobenzaldehyde with tribromomethane in dioxane with an aqueous solution of potassium hydroxide (Scheme 4).[24] Formation of methyl ester **22** was followed by an S_N2 displacement by thieno[3,2-*c*]pyridine (**20**) to afford [(±)-**1**] in 88% yield.

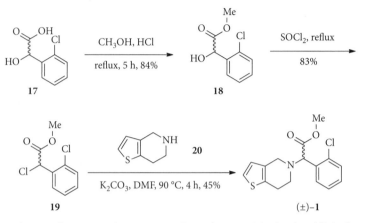

Scheme 3. The First Sanofi Discovery Synthesis of Racemic (±)-Clopidogrel [(±)–**1**]

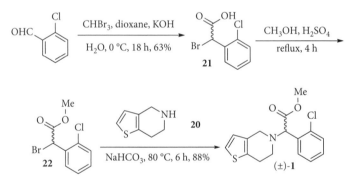

Scheme 4. The Second Sanofi Discovery Synthesis of Racemic (±)-Clopidogrel [(±)–**1**]

The individual enantiomers (+)-(**1**) and (–)-(**1**) were obtained from recrystallization of the diastereomers formed from (±)-**1** and levorotary camphor-10-sulfonic acid (see Scheme 5).

3.2 Process Route

With regard to the enantiomerically pure (+)-clopidogrel (**1**), it was originally obtained from resolution of the racemic clopidogrel [(±)-**1**] or through intermediates that were derived via resolution. For instance, racemic clopidogrel [(±)-**1**] was treated with levorotary camphor-10-sulfonic acid in acetone to afford salt **23**, which was recrystallized from acetone to generate (+)-clopidogrel (**1**, Scheme 5).[25]

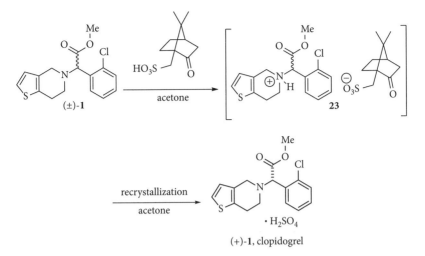

Scheme 5. The Sanofi Preparation of Enantiomerically Pure (+)-Clopidogrel (1)

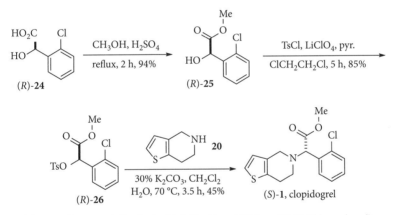

Scheme 6. Asymmetric Synthesis of (+)-Clopidogrel (1) from (R)-(2-Chloro-phenyl)-
hydroxy-acetic Acid (24)

One Sanofi synthesis of enantiomerically pure (+)-clopidogrel (1) utilized optically pure (R)-(2-chloro-phenyl)-hydroxy-acetic acid (24), a mandelic acid derivative, available from a chiral pool (Scheme 6).[26] After formation of methyl ester
(R)-25, tosylation of (R)-25 using toluenesulfonyl chloride led to α-tolenesulfonate
ester (R)-26. Subsequently, the S$_N$2 displacement of (R)-26 with thieno[3,2-c]pyr-
idine (20) then constructed (+)-clopidogrel (1).

Another Sanofi process synthesis of enantiomerically pure (+)-clopidogrel (1)
took advantage of resolution of racemic α-amino acid (±)-27 to access (S)-27 (Scheme
7).[27] The methyl ester 28 was prepared by treatment of (S)-27 with thionyl chloride
and methanol. Subsequent S$_N$2 displacement of (2-thienyl)-ethyl para-toluene-sulfo-
nate (29) with 28 assembled amine 30. Finally, ring-closure was achieved by heating
30 with paraformaldehyde in formic acid at reflux to give (+)-clopidogrel (1).

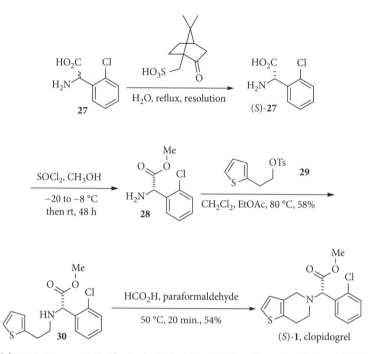

Scheme 7. Asymmetric Synthesis of (+)-Clopidogrel (**1**) from Racemic α-Amino Acid **27**

3.3 Synthesis of Radio-labeled API

A synthesis of labeled (±)-clopidogrel [(±)-**1**] has been described (Scheme 8).[28] The synthesis commenced with commercially available [*benzene*-U-^{13}C]-benzoic acid (**31**). Treating the acid chloride of **31** with 2-amino-2-methyl-propan-1-ol gave the corresponding amide, which was subsequently treated with thionyl chloride to afford oxazoline **32**. Applying Meyers' oxazoline-directed *ortho*-lithiation methodology, **32** was exposed to *s*-butyllithium and then quenched with hexachloroethane to give chloride **33** in 60% yield after separation of unreacted starting material **32**. Methylation of oxazoline **33** was followed by reduction of the resulting iminium intermediate to give trimethyl-oxazolidine **34**. Acidic hydrolysis of the cyclic hemiaminal functionality on **34** then produced [*benzene*-U-^{13}C]-2-chlorobenzaldehyde (**35**). A Strecker reaction on aldehyde **35** with 4,5,6,7-tetra-hydro-thieno[3,2-*c*]pyridine (**20**) in the presence of acetone cyanohydrin and $MgSO_4$ in toluene assembled nitrile **36**. While saponification of **36** under strong basic conditions resulted in, predominantly, a retro-Strecker reaction, hydro-chloric acid-promoted hydrolysis gave primary amide **37** in nearly quantitative yield. Finally, methanolysis and salt formation proceeded uneventfully to deliver [*benzene*-U-^{13}C]-(±)-clopidogrel [(±)-**1**]. The overall yield for this sequence from [*benzene*-U-^{13}C]-benzoic acid (**31**) to [*benzene*-U-^{13}C]-(±)-clopidogrel [(±)-**1**] was 7%.

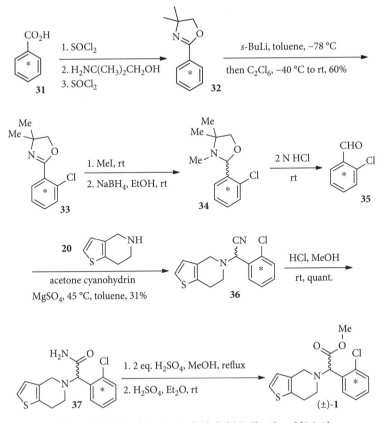

Scheme 8. The Sanofi Synthesis of Labeled (±)-Clopidogrel [(±)-1]

■ 4 CONCLUDING REMARKS

In 2009, the FDA approved prasugrel (**38**, Effient) for the reduction of thrombotic cardiovascular events (including stent thrombosis) in patients with ACS who are managed with an artery-opening procedure known as percutaneous coronary intervention (PCI).[29] But Effient has to carry a black box warning about its potential for "significant, sometimes fatal, bleeding." Effient is the third generation thienopyridine blood thinner developed by Eli Lilly and Daiichi Sankyo, Japan's largest pharmaceutical company. Daiichi Sankyo came up with prasugrel by modifying clopidogrel's structure. The key difference is that prasugrel has a ketone group to replace clopidogrel's methyl ester. As a consequence in vivo prasugrel does not have the acid metabolite, which is inactive in antiplatelet aggregation.

Because Plavix and Effient, both thienopyridines, are ADP-dependent platelet aggregation inhibitors, efforts are ongoing to find inhibitors that are not thienopyridines.

AstraZeneca's ticagrelor (**39**, Brilinta) is the fruit of such endeavors. Like Plavix and Effient, Brilinta blocks ADP receptors of subtype P2Y$_{12}$. Unlike Plavix and Effient, Brilinta's platelet aggregation inhibition activity is reversible. Moreover, it does not need hepatic activation, which could reduce the risk of DDI.[30] In July 2011, the FDA approved ticagrelor (**39**, Brilinta) for marketing in the United States.

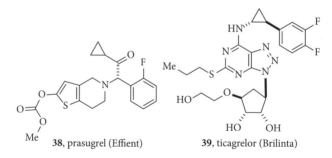

38, prasugrel (Effient)   **39**, ticagrelor (Brilinta)

Both fondaparinux (**2**) and idraparinux (**3**) are selective *indirect* factor Xa inhibitors which act through reversible high affinity binding to antithrombin, with very little effect on platelet aggregation. Factor Xa is a trypsin-like serine protease that plays an essential role in the coagulation cascade. Given its importance, *oral* factor Xa inhibitors would be better anticoagulants and the pharmaceutical industry has been hard at work to find them for the last decades.

The first oral factor Xa inhibitor, approved by the FDA in 2011, was Bayer's rivaroxaban (**40**, Xarelto).[31] The second oral factor Xa inhibitor, approved by the FDA in 2012, was Bristol-Myers Squibb's apixaban (**41**, Eliquis).[32]

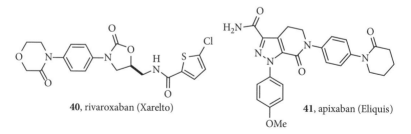

40, rivaroxaban (Xarelto)   **41**, apixaban (Eliquis)

Boehringer-Ingelheim's, dabigatran etexilate (**42**, Pradaxa), a direct thrombin inhibitor, was approved by the FDA in 2011.[33]

These oral anticoagulants may provide patients more options in selecting their appropriate treatments.

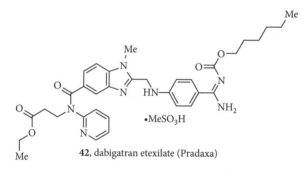

42, dabigatran etexilate (Pradaxa)

■ 5 REFERENCES

1. Marcum, J. A. *J. Hist. Med. Allied Sci.* **2000**, *55*, 37–66.

2. Messamore, H. L., Jr.; Wehrmacher, W. H.; Coyne, E. C.; Fareed, J. *Semin. Thromb. Hemost.* **2004**, *30(Suppl. 1)*, 81–88.

3. Griminger, P. *J. Nutrition* **1986**, *117*, 1325–1329.

4. Duxbury, B. M.; Poller, L. *Clin. Appl. Thromb.* **2001**, *7*, 269–275.

5. Kresge, N; Simoni, R. D.; Hill, R. L. *J. Biol. Chem.* **2005**, *280*, e5–e6.

6. Pirmohamed M. *Br. J. Clin. Pharmacol.* **2006**, *62*, 509–511.

7. Weiss, H. J. *J. Thromb. Haemost.* **2003**, *1*, 1869–1875.

8. Vane, J. R.; Botting, R. M. *Thromb Res.* **2003**, *110*, 255–258.

9. Gustafsson D. *Semin. Vasc. Med.* **2005**, *5*, 227–234.

10. Gurewich, V. *JAMA* **2005**, *293*, 736–739.

11. Maffrand, J. P.; Eloy, F. *Eur. J. Med. Chem.* **1974**, *9*, 483–486.

12. Ticlopidine, (a) Saltiel, E.; Ward, A. *Drugs* **1987**, *100*, 1667–1672. (b) Castañer, J. *Drugs Fut.* **1976**, *1*, 190–193. (c) Steinhubl, S. R.; Tan, W. A.; Foody, J. M.; Topol, E. J. *JAMA* **1999**, *281*, 806–810.

13. Jarvis, B.; Simpson, K. *Drugs* **2000**, *60*, 347–377.

14. Herbert, J. M.; Fréhel, D.; Bernat, A.; Badorc, A.; Savi, P.; Delebasseee, D.; Kieffer, G.; Defreyn, G.; Maffrand, J. P. *Drugs Fut.* **1996**, *21*, 1017–1021.

15. Escolar, G.; Heras, M. *Drugs Today* **2000**, *36*, 187–199.

16. Pereillo, J. M.; Maftouh, M.; Andrieu, A.; Uzabiaga, M.-F.; Fedeli, O.; Savi, O.; Pascal, M.; Herbert, J.-M.; Maffrand, J. P.; Picard, C. *Drug Metab. Dispos.* **2002**, *30*, 1288–1295.

17. MOA of Ticlopidine and Clopidogrel, Savi, P.; Labouret, C.; Delesque, N.; Guette, F.; Lupker, H.; Herbert, J. M. *Biochem. Biophysic. Res. Commun.* **2001**, *283*, 379–383.

18. Farid, N. A.; Kurihara, A.; Wrighton, S. A. *J. Clin. Pharmacol.* **2010**, *50*, 126–142.

19. Pare, G.; Mehta, S. R.; Yusuf, S.; Anand, S. S.; Connolly, S. J.; Hirsh, J.; Simonsen, K.; Bhatt, D. L.; Fox, K. A. A.; Eikelboom, J. W. *New Engl. J. Med.* **2010**, *363*, 1704–1714.

20. Cattaneo, M. *Eur. Heart J. Suppl.* **2008**, *10(Suppl I)*, I33–I37. Permission granted.

21. Rosenblum, S. B. Advances in the Development of Methods for the Synthesis of Cholesterol Absorption Inhibitors [Ezetimibe (Zetia, Ezetrol)], in *Art of Drug Synthesis* Johnson, D. S.; Li, J. J., Eds.; Wiley: Hoboken, NJ, 2007, pp. 183–196.

22. Stein, Sidney H., U.S.D.J., United States District Court Southern District of New York *Opinion and Order, 02 Civ. 2255 (SHS), Sanofi-Synthelabo; Sanofi-Synthelabo, Inc.; and Bristol-Myers Squibb Sanofi Pharmaceuticals Holding Partnership, Plaintiffs, against Apotex Inc. and Apotex Corp.;* June 19, 2007, New York.

23. Maffrand, J. P.; Eloy, F. *Eur. J. Med. Chem.* **1974**, *9*, 483–486.

24. Maffrand, J. P.; Eloy, F. *J. Heterocycl. Chem.* **1976**, *13*, 1347–1349.

25. Badorc, A.; Fréhel, D. *Dextro-rotatory Enantiomer of Methyl a-5-(4,5,6,7-Tetrahydro (3,2-c)ThienoPyridyl)(2-Chlorophenyl)-Acetate and The Pharmaceutical Compositions Containing It.* US 48747265 (1989).

26. (a) Bouisset, M.; Radison, J. US 5036156 (1991). (b) Bousquet, A.; Musolino, A. *Hydroxyacetic Ester Derivatives, Preparation Method and Use as Synthesis Intermediates,* WO 9918110 (1999).

27. (a) Braye, E. *Process for the Preparation of Thieno-Pyridine Derivatives,* US 4127580 (1977). (b) Descamps, M.; Radisson, J. *Process for The Preparation of an N-Phenylacetic Derivative of Tetrahydrothieno(3,2-c)Pyridine and Its Chemical Intermediate* US 5204469 (1993). (c) Aubert, D.; Ferrand, C.; Maffrand, J.-P. US 4529596 (1985).

28. Burgos, A.; Herbert, J. M.; Simpson, I. *J Labelled Compd. Radiopharm.* **2000**, *43*, 891–898.

29. Angiolillo, D. J.; Suryadevara, S.; Capranzano, P.; Bass, T. A. Prasugrel: *Exp Opin Pharmacother* **2008**, *9*, 2893–2900.

30. Deeks, E. D. *Drugs* **2011**, *71*, 909–933.

31. Roehrig, S.; Straub, A.; Pohlmann, J.; Lampe, T.; Pernerstorfer, J.; Schlemmer, K.-H.; Reinemer, P.; Perzborn, E. *J. Med. Chem.* **2005**, *48*, 5900–5908.

32. Pinto, D. J. P.; Orwat, M. J.; Koch, S. et al. *J. Med. Chem.* **2007**, *50*, 5339–5356.

33. Eriksson, B. I.; Smith, H.; Yasothan, U.; Kirkpatrick, P. *Nat. Rev. Drug Discov.* **2008**, *7*, 557–558.

3   Amlodipine (Novasc)

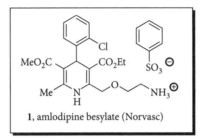

1, amlodipine besylate (Norvasc)

USAN:	*Amlodipine Besylate*
Brand Name:	*Norvasc (Pfizer)*
Molecular Weight:	*567.06 (Parent 408.88)*
FDA Approval:	*1990*
Drug Class:	*1,4-Dihydropyridine Calcium Channel Blocker*
Indications:	*Treatment of Hypertension and Angina Pectoris*
Mechanism of Action:	*Calcium Channel Blocker (Inhibition of the Trans-membrane Influx of Calcium Ions into Vascular Smooth Muscle and Cardiac Muscle with Peripheral Arterial Vasodilatation)*

■ 1 HISTORY

Hypertension (high blood pressure) is estimated to afflict 1 billion individuals worldwide and is a major risk factor for stroke, coronary artery disease, heart failure, and end-stage renal disease.[1] The first class of drugs to treat hypertension was the mercurial diuretics, discovered by Alfred Vogl in 1919 in Vienna.[2] Diuretics, by removing fluid from the body, reduce the pressure on the heart. Mercurial diuretics revolutionized the treatment of congestive heart failure resulting from severe edema and were the primary treatment until the late 1950s, when thiazide diuretics emerged. In 1957, Merck chemist Frederick C. Novello prepared chlorothiazide (**2**, Diuril), a potent diuretic that does not cause elevation of bicarbonate excretion, an undesired side effect associated with mercurial diuretics.[3] Shortly after chlorothiazide's (**2**) success, George deStevens at Ciba reduced a double bond on chlorothiazide (**2**) to a single bond to give hydrochlorothiazide (**3**, HydroDiuril) which was 10-fold more potent than the prototype **2**.[4] Hydrochlorothiazide was introduced to medical practice in 1959 and within a short time became the drug of choice for the treatment of mild hypertension.

One of the liabilities of these drugs is thiazide diuretic-induced hyperglycemia.

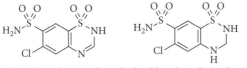

2, chlorothiazide (Diuril) **3**, hydrochlorothiazide (HydroDiuril)

As early as 1948, Raymond P. Ahlquist at the Medical College of Georgia speculated that there were two types of adrenergic receptors (adrenoceptors in short),
which he termed α-adrenoceptor and β-adrenoceptor, that are 7-transmembraned
protein as GPCR.[5] In 1957, Irwin H. Slater and C. E. Powell at Eli Lilly prepared
dichloroisoprenaline (DCI, **4**), the dichloro analog of isoprenaline; it was later
found to be the first selective β-adrenoreceptor blocking reagent, also known as a
β-blocker. However, DCI was not further pursued as a drug candidate because it
had a marked undesirable stimulant effect on the heart, an intrinsic sympathomimetic action (ISA).[6] Beginning in 1958, James Black at Imperial Chemical Industries (ICI) led a team to look for β-blockers that were devoid of the stimulant effect
on the heart. In 1962, the first selective β-adrenoreceptor inhibitor pronethalol (**5**)
was discovered but was withdrawn from further development when it was found
to cause thymic tumors in mice. ICI eventually in 1964 produced a drug propranolol (**6**, Inderal), which possessed a better efficacy and safety profile.[7] Propranolol
(**6**) is now widely used in the management of angina, hypertension, arrhythmia,
and migraine headaches. Two additional β-blockers, atenolol (Tenormin) and
practolol (Dalzic), were later discovered and marketed by ICI. Dozens of "me-too"
selective beta-blockers have since been discovered and marketed.

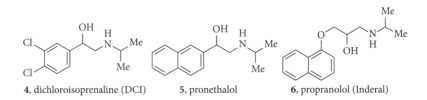

4, dichloroisoprenaline (DCI)   **5**, pronethalol   **6**, propranolol (Inderal)

Angiotensin converting enzyme (ACE) inhibitors are widely used to treat hypertension, congestive heart failure, and heart attacks. The MOA of ACE inhibitors is through inhibiting ACE in the renin–angiotensin system (RAS), which is
the master regulator of blood pressure and cardiovascular function. RAS provided
numerous targets for pharmacologic intervention (Fig. 3.1).[11] Although renin catalyzes the first and rate-limiting step (see **12** below) in the activation of the RAS, it
was the inhibition of the downstream ACE that first established the clinical rele-
vance of this pathway in the treatment of hypertension.

David Cushman and Miguel A. Ondetti at the Squibb Institute isolated teprotide, a nonapeptide, from the poisonous venom extract of the Brazilian pit viper

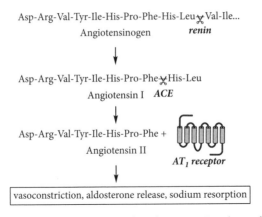

Asp-Arg-Val-Tyr-Ile-His-Pro-Phe-His-Leu—Val-Ile...
Angiotensinogen   *renin*

Asp-Arg-Val-Tyr-Ile-His-Pro-Phe—His-Leu
Angiotensin I   *ACE*

Asp-Arg-Val-Tyr-Ile-His-Pro-Phe +
Angiotensin II

AT₁ receptor

| vasoconstriction, aldosterone release, sodium resorption |

Fig. 3.1. The Renin–Angiotensin System (RAS) as the Master Regulator of Blood Pressure[11]

Bothrops jararaca. Using teprotide, a potent ACE inhibitor in vitro, as a starting point, Cushman and Ondetti curtailed the molecule, replaced its carboxylate group with a thiol (–SH), and achieved a 2,000-fold increase in potency in ACE inhibition. The resulting drug became the first *oral* ACE inhibitor, captopril (**7**, Capoten).[8] Merck scientists led by Arthur A. Patchett discovered the second oral ACE inhibitor, enalapril (**8**, Vasotec), which has been on the market since 1981.[9] Another popular ACE inhibitor is Parke-Davis's quinapril hydrochloride (**9**, Accupril), launched in 1991.[10]

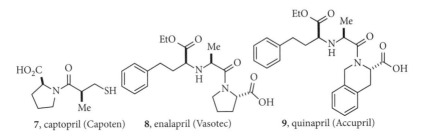

7, captopril (Capoten)   8, enalapril (Vasotec)   9, quinapril (Accupril)

Also as shown in Fig. 3.1, angiotensin II is a potent vasoconstrictor; blocking its action would result in vasodilation. DuPont-Merck Pharmaceuticals discovered the first inhibitor of the angiotensin II receptor, losartan (**10**, Cozaar), which after its launch in 1995 quickly became one of the most important drugs for the treatment of high blood pressure.[12] Other angiotensin II receptor antagonists (also known as angiotensin receptor blockers, or ARBs) include Novartis's valsartan (**11**, Diovan),[12] Sanofi-Aventis's irbesartan (Avapro), AstraZeneca's candesartan (Atacand), and Boehringer-Ingelheim's telmisartan (Micardis). They all proved to be superior to ACE inhibitors because they did not cause the irritating cough that occurs in a small percentage of patients taking ACE inhibitors.

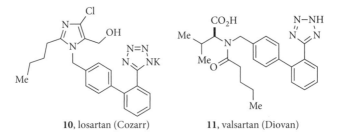

10, losartan (Cozarr)   **11**, valsartan (Diovan)

Since renin is extremely specific for angiotensinogen and is the first and rate-limiting enzyme of the RAS, renin inhibition was recognized for decades as an attractive approach for the treatment of hypertension and hypertension-related target organ damage. Novartis's aliskiren (**12**, Tekturna) is the first and the only renin inhibitor on the market for treatment of hypertension, and has been since 2007.[11]

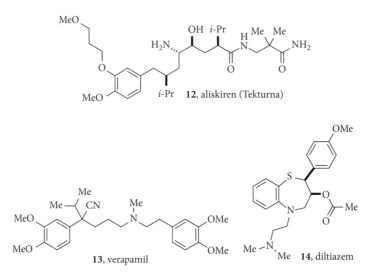

12, aliskiren (Tekturna)

13, verapamil   **14**, diltiazem

The concept of calcium channel blockers (CCBs), also known as calcium channel antagonists or calcium entry blockers, was developed several years *after* some CCBs including phenylalkylamines such as verapamil (**13**), perhexiline, and prenylamine; and benzodiazepines such as diltiazem (**14**) were discovered. Albrecht Fleckenstein at University of Freiburg in Germany and Winifred G. Nayler helped to elucidate the mechanism of action (MOA) of those structurally diversified drugs as CCBs.[13]

In 1969, Bayer Company investigated the pharmacology of Bay-a-1040 (**15**, nifedipine) and Bay-a-7168 (niludipine). Both compounds were strong coronary vasodilators and exerted significant negative inotropic effects on the myocardium. With Fleckenstein's help, Bayer elucidated their MOA as CCBs. Nifedipine (**15**,

Adalat) heralded the beginning of one of the most important classes of calcium antagonists: 1,4-dihydropyridines.[13]

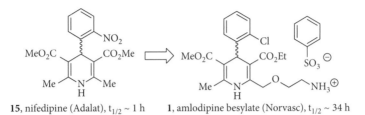

15, nifedipine (Adalat), $t_{1/2} \sim 1$ h   **1**, amlodipine besylate (Norvasc), $t_{1/2} \sim 34$ h

Bayer's nifedipine (**15**, Adalat), known as a first-generation CCB, is a short-acting CCB with a short plasma half-life (in the range of 0.5 to 2 h). Therefore, Adalat has to be taken 3 or 4 times a day to elicit 24-h blood pressure control. Efforts to improve bioavailability resulted in the second-generation CCBs, including isradipine ($t_{1/2} \sim 2$ h), nicardipine ($t_{1/2}, \sim 5$ h), and felodipine ($t_{1/2}, \sim 10$ h). Pfizer's amlodipine (**1**, Norvasc), launched in 1990, belongs to the third-generation of CCBs. It has a high bioavailability (64%) and a longer half-life (~45 h) in plasma, so it can be taken once daily.[14] All of these features made amlodipine (**1**, Norvasc) the most prescribed antihypertensive agent in the world in 2003 with an annual sale of $4.3 billion. The worldwide sales of calcium channel blockers totaled $6 billion that year.

■ 2 PHARMACOLOGY

2.1 Mechanism of Action

Inside a normal cell, the concentration of free Ca^{2+} ions is low (10^{-7} M) in comparison to that of the extracellular fluid (1–2 mM). The concentration may be regulated by opening or closing of the calcium channels. Calcium channels are opened temporarily by exogenous impulses, whereby the calcium ion concentration rises briefly and Ca^{2+} ions are bound to calcium-binding proteins (calmodulin). The activated calmodulin elicits actual reactions in the cell and the increased calcium concentration is reduced rapidly to the initial value by uptake of Ca^{2+} ions into intracellular reserves.

The calcium channel, located on the cell membrane, is an ion channel that is selectively permeable to calcium ions (Fig. 3.2). Since the results of calcium ions entering the cell membrane include contraction of smooth muscle cells, blocking the entrance of calcium ions into the cell would result in vasodilation, thus lowering the blood pressure. When a CCB enters the opening of a calcium channel, the drug figuratively gets stuck, like a fat man caught halfway through a porthole, thus preventing calcium ions from getting through the channel.

Amlodipine (**1**, Norvasc) and other CCBs inhibit the influx of Ca^{2+} ions into cells without affecting inward Na^+ or outward K^+ currents to a significant degree.

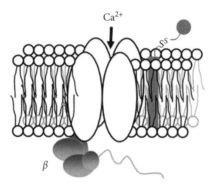

Fig. 3.2. The Calcium Channel

The sizes of Ca^{2+}, Na^+, and K^+ are quite different so selectivity might be relatively easier to achieve if the drug is not too small.

Amlodipine acts by relaxing the smooth muscle in the arterial wall, decreasing total peripheral resistance and hence reducing blood pressure; in angina, it increases blood flow to the heart muscle. In vitro, amlodipine (**1**) inhibits Ca^{2+}-induced contractions of depolarized rat aorta with an IC_{50} of 1.9 nM, which is twice as potent as nifedipine (**15**, IC_{50} of 4.1 nM).[16]

Calcium channel blockers selectively slow or block the movement of the calcium ion into muscle cells via L-type voltage-gated calcium channels. The selectivity of their pharmacological effects appears to arise in particular because of the abundance of L channels in cardiac and smooth muscle. Dihydropyridines such as amlodipine (**1**) may also inhibit cyclic nucleotide phosphodiesterases (PDE). The dual capacity of the dihydropyridines to decrease cytosolic Ca^{2+} and to increase extracellular Ca^{2+} may contribute to their greater effects on vascular relaxation.

2.2 Structure–Activity Relationship

The structure–activity relationship (SAR) of the 1,4-dihydropyridines as CCBs has been extensively investigated.[17] As shown in Fig. 3.3, the NH group is critical to its activity, which is present on all 1,4-dihydropyridine CCBs. The R group at the C-2 position is alkyl (mostly methyl) in the majority of first- and second-generation 1,4-dihydropyridine CCBs. Amlodipine (**1**) carries a basic amine (pK_a, 8.6) group at the C-2 position, which is likely to contribute to its long half-life (~45 h) as well as its high bioavailability (64%). The ester function at the C-3 position seems to be able to accommodate a large variety of esters, α,β-unsaturated esters, and long-chain esters with bulky groups. As far as the C-4 aryl substitution is concerned, the *o*-group apparently prefers to be electron-withdrawing, as exemplified by the –Cl on amlodipine (**1**) and the $-NO_2$ on nifedipine (**15**). In addition, a fused bicyclic aryl group is also tolerated as exemplified by isradipine (not shown) with its benzo[*c*][1,2,5]oxadiazole group. Finally, the ester function at C-5 seems to be optimal in comparison to ketones, nitrile, and proton.

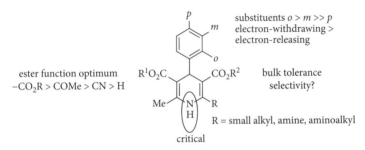

substituents $o > m >> p$
electron-withdrawing >
electron-releasing

ester function optimum
$-CO_2R > COMe > CN > H$

bulk tolerance
selectivity?

R = small alkyl, amine, aminoalkyl

critical

Fig. 3.3. The Structure–Activity Relationship (SAR) of the 1,4-Dihydropyridines

Like most of the newer CCBs, amlodipine (**1**) also has two different ester substituents and thus is sold as a mixture of isomers. Initial work on the analysis of the 2 possible isomers suggested that the R isomer (+)-**1** was more potent than the corresponding S isomer (–)-**1**; this suggested that amlodipine (**1**) differs in this respect from other dihydropyridine CCBs in which the S isomer is usually the more active. A more recent preparation of the (–)-(1S)-camphanic derivatives of amlodipine (**1**) and the subsequent X-ray of its derivatives clearly showed that it is the S derivative that is more active.[18]

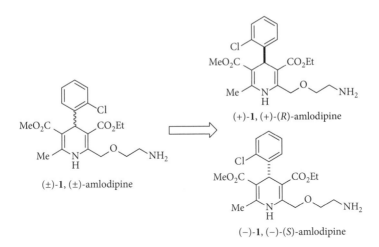

(±)-**1**, (±)-amlodipine

(+)-**1**, (+)-(R)-amlodipine

(–)-**1**, (–)-(S)-amlodipine

2.3 Bioavailability, Metabolism, and Toxicology

One unique feature of amlodipine (**1**) is that its 1,4-dihydropyridine ring carries a basic amine (pK_a, 8.6) group at the C-2 position. This renders the molecule >90% ionized at physiologic pH, and this feature is believed to be primarily responsible for the marked difference in physicochemical and pharmacokinetic properties displayed by amlodipine (**1**) as compared to other 1,4-dihydropyridines.

Initial evaluation of amlodipine (**1**) pharmacokinetics in dogs, mice, and rats indicated absolute bioavailability of 88%, 100%, and 100%, respectively.[19] Their corresponding calculated half-lives are 30 h, 11 h, and 3 h, respectively.

Single-dose pharmacokinetics in healthy male subjects after 10-mg intravenous injection indicated clearance of 7 mL/min/kg, volume of distribution by the area method of 21 L/kg, and calculated elimination half-life of 34 h. Absolute bioavailability of amlodipine (1) was determined by comparison of a single 10-mg oral dose (the highest dosage approved by the FDA) to the intravenous dose and was estimated to be 64%.[20]

Amlodipine (1) shows a preference for binding vascular smooth muscle cells over cardiac muscle cells, thus acting as a peripheral arterial vasodilator. Like most other CCB dihydropyridines, amlodipine (1) is highly protein-bound (98%) and heavily metabolized. In contrast to felodipine, amlodipine (1) is not influenced by grapefruit juice and appears to show fewer DDI.[21]

The major metabolic pathway for amlodipine (1) is oxidation by CYP450 to the corresponding pyridine 16, which is not active. All 1,4-dihydropyridines undergo similar metabolism to produce inactive pyridyl metabolites.[22]

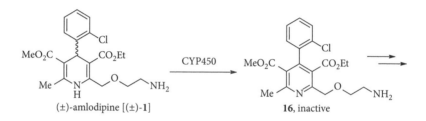

(±)-amlodipine [(±)-1]   16, inactive

Besides being effective on left ventricular hypertrophy, CCBs in general appear to be beneficial in slowing the progression of carotid hypertrophy and atherosclerosis. They are widely used in the treatment of high blood pressure, angina and rapid heartbeat (tachycardia) including arterial fibrillation.

The long duration of action makes amlodipine ideal for long-term treatment of hypertension. Moreover, it is safe and gradually reduces blood pressure. This is a good attribute, because reducing blood pressure too quickly can cause fainting spells, which happens with some of the 1,4-dihydropyridine calcium antagonists.

The adverse effects reported with amlodipine (1) are peripheral edema in 8.3% of users; fatigue in 4.5% of users; dizziness, palpitations, muscle-, stomach-, or headache, dyspepsia, and nausea in 1% of users.[23] Amlodipine (1) is contraindicated in breast feeding women and in patients with cardiogenic shock, unstable angina, and aortic stenosis, because amlodipine (1) causes vasodilatation which can result in reduced cardiac output in patients with severe aortic stenosis.

■ 3 SYNTHESIS

3.1 Discovery Route

The discovery synthesis of amlodipine (1) is outlined in Scheme 1, whose key step is a Hantzsch condensation of three-components.[17,18, 23]

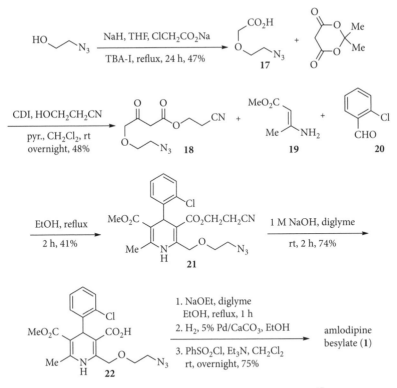

Scheme 1. Discovery Synthesis of Amlodipine Besylate (**1**)[17]

An S_N2 displacement of sodium chloroacetate with sodium azidoethoxide was accomplished with the aid of tetrabutylammonium iodide (TBA-I) as a phase-transfer catalyst (PTC) to afford (2-azidoethoxy)acetic acid (**17**). Esterification of acid **17** with 3-hydroxypropionitrile was helped with Meldrun's acid to give ester **18**. The crucial Hantzsch condensation of ester **18** with (*E*)-methyl 3-aminobut-2-enoate **19** and *o*-chlorobenzaldehyde (**20**) delivered 1,4-dihydropyridine **21**. After hydrolysis of ester **21** with 1 N NaOH to give acid **22**, treatment of **22** with NaOEt afforded the ethyl ester, which was hydrogenized to the corresponding amine using catalytic palladium on calcium carbonate or zinc and acetic acid. A number of salts of amlodipine (**1**) have been prepared, but the final commercial compound was obtained by treating the intermediate amine with benzenesulfonic chloride to prepare the corresponding besylate salt (**1**).[24]

3.2 Process Route

One of Pfizer's process preparations of amlodipine (**1**) is outlined in Scheme 2.[23–26] In this case, methyl-2-(2-chlorobenzylidene)acetoacetate (**25**) was prepared via

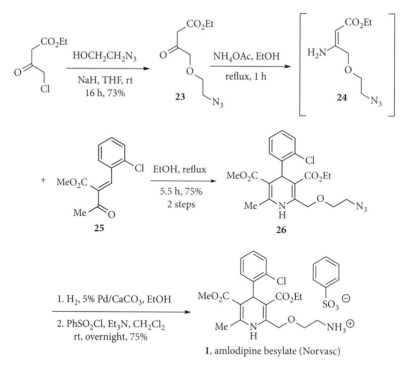

Scheme 2. Pfizer Process Synthesis of Amlodipine Besylate (1)[23]

Knoevenagel condensation of methyl acetoacetate and 2-chlorobenzaldehyde. Meanwhile, ethyl-4-(2-azidoethoxy)acetoacetate (23) was prepared via an S_N2 reaction from the sodium salt of 2-azidoethanol and ethyl-4-chloroacetoacetate. Intermediate azide 23 was then treated with ammonium acetate to give enamine 24. The Hantzsch condensation of 24 with Knoevenagel adduct 25 then furnished the dihydropyridine 26. After recrystallization, the azide functionality of 26 was reduced to the corresponding amine by using hydrogen and catalytic palladium on calcium carbonate or zinc and acetic acid to give the intermediate amine, which was treated with benzenesulfonic acid to prepare the corresponding besylate salt 1.[23]

To overcome the real or the perceived safety issues associated with azide intermediates, an alternative process route not involving azide was explored.[25]

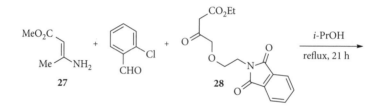

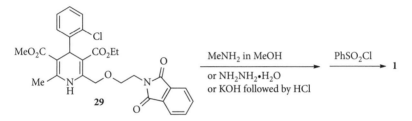

Scheme 3. Pfizer Process Synthesis of Amlodipine Besylate (**1**)[25]

■ 4 CONCLUDING REMARKS

The last 50 years saw tremendous advances in the number of treatments available for managing hypertension, angina, and related coronary artery diseases: diuretics, beta-blockers, ACE inhibitors, ARBs, renin inhibitor, and CCBs. Among CCBs, amlodipine (**1**, Norvasc) and other long-acting 1,4-dihydropyridines have the additional advantage of only requiring a once-daily dosing regimen.

Unfortunately, despite the availability of a wide range of antihypertensive medications, about 45.5% of treated patients in the US fail to achieve a blood pressure control target of <140/90 mmHg. Since the detrimental ramifications of hypertension include damage to the arteries, heart, kidneys, and brain, there is still a large unmet medical need in the field of antihypertensives. One recent trend is the combination pill. For instance, Pfizer combined amlodipine (**1**, Norvasc) with atorvastatin (Lipitor, see Chapter 1) and sold it as one pill under the trade name Caduet.

■ 5 REFERENCES

1. (a) Mancia, G.; Grassi, G. *J. Hypertens. Suppl.* **1998**, *16*, S1–S7. (b) Prichard, B. N. *Drugs* **1988**, *35*(Suppl 6), 40–52.

2. Vogl, A. *Am. Heart. J.* **1950**, *39*, 881–883.

3. Beyer, K. H. *Persp. Biol. Med.* **1977**, *20*, 410–420.

4. deStevens, G. *J. Med. Chem.* **1991**, *34*, 2665–2670.

5. Ahlquist, Raymond P. *Ann. Rev. Pharmacol.* **1968**, *8*, 259–272.

6. Powell, C. E.; Slater, I. H.; LeCompte, L., Jr.; Waddell, J. E. *J. Pharmacol. Exp. Ther.* **1958**, *122*, 480–488.

7. Crowther, A. F. *Drug Des. Deliv.* **1990**, *6*, 149–156.

8. Smith, C. G.; Vane, J. R. *FASEB J.* **2003**, *17*, 788–789.

9. Patchett, A. A. *J. Med. Chem.* **2002**, *45*, 5609–5616.

10. Klutchko, S.; Blankley, C. J.; Fleming, R. W. et al. *J. Med. Chem.* **1986**, *29*, 1953–1961.

11. Cee, V. in *Modern Drug Synthesis*, Li, J. J.; Johnson, D. S., Eds, Wiley: Hoboken, NJ 2010, pp. 141–158.

12. Yet, L. Advances in the development of methods for the synthesis of antihypertensive drugs (angiotensin At1 antagonists) in *The Art of Drug Synthesis*, Johnson, D. S.; Li, J. J., Eds, Wiley: Hoboken, NJ, 2007, pp. 129–141.

13. (a) Fleckenstein-Grün, G. *High Blood Pressure*, **1994**, *3*, 284–290. (b) Goldmann, S. *Pharmazie* **2005**, *34*, 366–373.

14. Epstein, B. J.; Vogel, K.; Palmer, B. F. *Drugs* **2007**, *67*, 1309–1327.

15. Hanlon, M. R.; Berrow, N. S.; Dolphin, A. C.; Wallace, B. A. *FEBS Lett.* **1999**, *445*, 366–370. Burges, R. A.; Dodd, M. G.; Gardiner, D. G. *Am. J. Cardiol.* **1989**, *64*, 10I–20I.

16. Triggle, D. J. Ion Channels, in *A Textbook of Drug Design and Development*, Krogsgaard-Larsen, P.; Bundgaard, H., Eds, Harwood Academic Publishers: Chur, Switzerland, 1991, pp. 357–386.

17. Arrowsmith, J. E.; Campbell, S. F.; Cross, P. E.; Stubbs, J. K.; Burges, R. A.; Gardiner, D. G.; Blackburn, K. J. *J. Med. Chem.* **1986**, *29*, 1696–1702.

18. Abernethy, D. R. *Am. Heart J.* **1989**, *118*, 1100–1103.

19. Murdoch, D.; Heel, R. C. *Drugs* **1991**, *41*, 478–505.

20. Josefsson, M.; Zackrisson, A. L.; Ahlner, J. *Eur. J. Clin. Pharmacol.* **1996**, *51*, 189–193.

21. Beresford, A. P.; McGibney, D.; Humphrey, M. J.; Macrae, P. V.; Stopher, D. A. *Xenobiotica* **1988**, *18*, 245–254.

22. Osterloh, I. H. *J. Cardiovas. Pharmacol.* **1991**, *17*(Suppl 1), S65–S68.

23. Davison, E.; Wells, J. I. (to Pfizer, Inc.). *Pharmaceutically Acceptable Salts*. US 4,879,303 (1989).

24. Campbell, S. F.; Cross, P. E.; Stubbs, J. K. (to Pfizer, Inc.). *Dihydropyridine Anti-Ischemic and Antihypertensive Agents and Pharmaceutical Compositions Containing Them* EP 89167 (1983).

25. Campbell, S. F.; Cross, P. E.; Stubbs, J. K. (to Pfizer, Inc.). *2-(Secondary Amino-alkoxymethyl)-Dihydropyridine Derivatives as Anti-Ischaemic and Antihypertensive Agents*. US 4,572,909 (1986).

Cancer Drugs

4   Paclitaxel (Taxol)

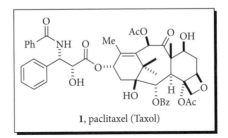

1, paclitaxel (Taxol)

USAN: *Paclitaxel*
Brand Name: *Taxol (Bristol-Myers Squibb)*
Molecular Weight: *839.92*
FDA Approval: *1992*
Drug Class: *Anticancer*
Indications: *Ovarian, Breast, and Non–Small-Cell Lung Cancer; Kaposi's Sarcoma*
Mechanism of Action: *Microtubule-stabilizing Agent (Tubulin Polymerization Agent)*

▪ 1 HISTORY

Cancer is a disease of cellular dysfunction involving a range of biological activities that promote unregulated proliferation. It is as old as the existence of animals—cancers are found even in dinosaur bones. Approximately 110 types of cancer have been characterized. In particular, breast cancer (second only to lung cancer in terms of fatality rate) strikes one in eight women and there are approximately 200,000 annual incidents in the United States alone. About 25% of women with breast carcinoma eventually will die from their disease. Genetic predisposition is largely blamed for the genesis of breast cancer, as well as colon and prostate cancers.

In terms of the genesis of cancer, the carcinogen theory emerged first. Carcinogens are agents such as chemicals, X-rays, and UV light that cause cancers. As early as 1775, British doctor Percival Pott made an astute epidemiological observation that young English boys employed as chimney sweeps were more prone to develop scrotal skin cancers than their French counterparts.[1] Further scrutiny revealed that the continental sweeps bathed more frequently after work, which prompted Pott to speculate that long exposure to coal tar caused skin cancer. Pott's theory was later confirmed experimentally by Katsusaburo Yamagiwa and Koichi

Ichikawa in Japan in 1914. Nowadays, the carcinogenicity of a compound is routinely screened using the Ames test.

In 1966, Peyton Rous at the Rockefeller Institute won the Nobel Prize in Physiology or Medicine for his discovery of tumor-inducing viruses. Fifty years previously in 1909, Rous was able to artificially produce for the first time a tumor in an animal (chicken) using a tumor virus, which was later named the Rous sarcoma virus, or RSV.[2] Viral infections have now been implicated—hepatic cancers are caused by hepatitis B or C viruses (HBV and HCV), cervical cancer is caused by papilloma virus, and T-cell leukemia is caused by human T-lymphotropic virus 1 (HTLV-1). In addition, the *Helicobacter pylori* bacterium infection is a major risk factor for stomach cancer. The past several decades saw wide acceptance of the oncogene theory,[3] but that is beyond the scope of this book.

The current arsenal of treatment for breast cancer includes surgery (i.e., mastectomy or lumpectomy), radiation, chemotherapy, and hormone treatment.

An aggressive chemotherapy[4] regimen typically includes cyclophosphamide (**2**, Cytoxan), 5-FU (**3**, fluorouracil), and methotrexate (**4**). Cytoxan (**2**) is a nitrogen mustard, an alkylating agent discovered in the 1940s. Alkylating agents kill both resting and multiplying cancer cells. Specifically, they work by interfering with the chemical growth processes of cancer cells, thus preventing DNA from uncoiling and thereby blocking DNA replication and cell division. Unfortunately, alkylating agents also destroy healthy cells indiscriminately. The use of such drugs has often been compared to a "carpet bombing" strategy. By the same mechanism, a common side effect to such cancer treatment is hair loss—alkylating agents also kill hair follicle cells along with active dividing cancer cells. On the other hand, 5-FU (**3**) and methotrexate (**4**), a folic acid analogue, are antimetabolites. They prevent cancer cells from metabolizing nutrients and other essential substances, thus blocking processes within the cell that lead to cell division.

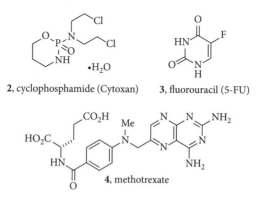

2, cyclophosphamide (Cytoxan)   **3**, fluorouracil (5-FU)

4, methotrexate

The female hormone (estrogen) can fuel the growth of breast cancer cells, and pregnancy should be avoided for breast cancer patients. Tamoxifen (**5**, Nolvadex) was initially developed by ICI as a birth-control pill. Although it was ineffective as a contraceptive in animal models, the FDA approved tamoxifen (**5**) for the treatment of metastatic breast cancer in 1977, and tamoxifen is now the most frequently prescribed anticancer drug in the world. It is a partial antagonist and partial agonist of the estrogen receptor (ER). It blocks the generation of estrogen in some parts of the body while acts like estrogen in some other parts of the body. More specifically, it is a SERM, that is, a selective estrogen receptor modulator. Tamoxifen (**5**) is very well tolerated but recently has been shown to lead sometimes to blood clots and endometrial cancer. Since estrogen is a key trigger in two-thirds of all breast cancers, after surgery, radiation and chemotherapy, the estrogen-dependent breast cancer patient is often treated with tamoxifen. In 1998, the FDA also approved tamoxifen for prophylactic use in women at high risk of developing breast cancer (those who have ER-positive tumors)—patients taking tamoxifen are 45% less likely to get breast cancer recurrence. However, because tamoxifen acts as a stimulant of estrogen action in the uterus and thus could cause uterine cancer, it is less desirable as a breast cancer preventive. A newer SERM, raloxifene (**6**, Evista)[5] renders a 58% reduction of breast cancer.

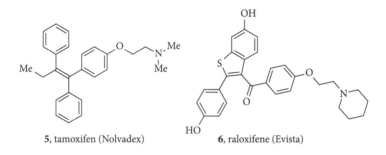

5, tamoxifen (Nolvadex)   **6**, raloxifene (Evista)

Despite the significant benefit that tamoxifen has bestowed on breast cancer patients, the third-generation aromatase inhibitors are rapidly replacing tamoxifen (**5**) as the first-line treatment for breast cancers. Aromatase is the enzyme (in body fat, the liver, and the adrenal glands) that converts androgen to estrogen. Aromatase inhibitors may be classified into three types. Type I aromatase inhibitors bind to the aromatase enzyme irreversibly, so they are called inactivators. In some cases they are dubbed mechanism-based or "suicide" inhibitors when they are metabolized by the enzyme into reactive intermediates that bind covalently to the active site. Type I aromatase inhibitors are usually steroidal in structure as represented by Pharmacia's exemestane (**7**, Aromasin), Novartis's formestane (**8**, Lentaron), and Schering's atamestane (**9**).[6]

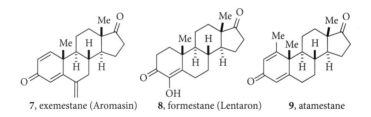

7, exemestane (Aromasin)   **8**, formestane (Lentaron)   **9**, atamestane

Type II aromatase inhibitors reversibly bind to the enzyme. The first Type II aromatase inhibitor marketed for the treatment of breast cancer was aminoglutethimide (**10**), marketed by Ciba-Geigy since 1981. Aminoglutethimide (**10**) is not very selective, binding to several steroidal hydroxylases that have the CYP prosthetic group. Thankfully, continued SAR development led to the latest type III aromatase inhibitors such as anastrozole (**11**) and letrozole (**12**) with exceptional specificity for the aromatase P450 enzyme. Therefore, there are fewer selectivity-related toxicities with the drugs. While formestane (**10**) is a Type II aromatase inhibitor, anastrozole (**11**) and letrozole (**12**) are considered Type III aromatase inhibitors.[6]

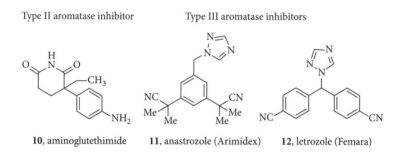

Type II aromatase inhibitor   Type III aromatase inhibitors

10, aminoglutethimide   **11**, anastrozole (Arimidex)   **12**, letrozole (Femara)

Paclitaxel (**1**, Taxol), has had considerable success in treating ovarian and breast cancer since 1992. It was initially isolated as part of the NCI-USDA (National Cancer Institute-United States Department of Agriculture) plant-screening program. In August 1962, Arthur Barclay at USDA traveled to the Gifford Pinchot Forest in Washington State and found a little known Pacific yew tree, *Taxus brevifolia*. He collected samples of twigs, leaves, and fruits, labeled them B-1046 and shipped them to the NCI.[7] After the cytotoxic effect of B-1046 extract was observed in 1966, Monroe E. Wall and Mansuhk C. Wani at the Research Triangle Institute took on the challenge to isolate and characterize the principal ingredient. Using bioactivity-directed fractionation, they were able to purify the crude extract so that the cytotoxic potency increased 1,000-fold. In 1967, they isolated the active principle as white crystals in a 0.014% yield from the dried bark of the Pacific yew. The molecule was later determined to have a molecular formula of $C_{47}H_{51}NO_4$ and a molecular weight of 839.[8] Wall christened the molecule "Taxol," where "tax" signified the origin of the molecule from *Taxus brevifolia*, and "ol" indicated that the molecule contained one or more alcohol functionalities.

Because of its insolubility, scarce supply, and low potency, there was no overwhelming enthusiasm for Taxol until 1979 when Susan Howitz,[9] an assistant professor at the Albert Einstein College of Medicine, discovered that Taxol had a completely novel MOA, unlike any other drug known at the time. It turns out that Taxol exerts its action by stabilizing the microtubules, resulting in inhibition of mitosis and induction of apoptosis. Taxol stops malignant tumors from growing by interfering with the microtubules that are responsible for dividing the chromosomes during cell division.

This novel mechanism rekindled interest in Taxol. The NCI took the torch from Wall, with Mathew Suffness as the champion. In 1984, the NCI amassed enough positive data to commence a phase I clinical trial of Taxol with about 30 patients. The drug was shown to be relatively safe. There was tremendous difficulty in procuring enough Taxol—it took about 20,000 lb of yew tree bark to isolate 1 kg of Taxol—but the NCI moved forward with the phase II trials in 1987. Taxol is notoriously insoluble in water but this was overcome by the addition of ethanol and Cremophor EL, a surfactant made of polyoxyethylated castor oil, which later proved to be important in reversing multidrug resistance. Although tested in ovarian cancer, renal cancer, and melanoma, Taxol initially was only found to be efficacious for ovarian cancer. Eventually, its chemotherapeutic applications were expanded to breast cancer, non–small-cell lung cancer, and Kaposi's sarcoma.[10]

Securing proof of concept (POC) from the phase II trial was a triumph for the NCI, which had overseen the clinical development of Taxol from the beginning, more than 20 years previously. However, the NCI was not equipped to take on the expensive and long phase III trials involving numerous disciplines such as oncology, pharmaceutical science, pharmacokinetics and drug metabolism, statistics, drug safety science, and others. Following a competitive selection process, Bristol-Myers Squibb (BMS), the only major US pharmaceutical company to have made a bid, was awarded the molecule under the Cooperative Research & Development Agreement (CRADA) with the NCI in 1991. At the time, the commercial potential of Taxol had not fully manifested for the breast cancer indication. The NCI's choice of BMS over the French company Rhône-Poulenc made sense because Rhône-Poulenc already had a competing—drug decetaxel (**14**, Taxotere) prepared from 10-deacetylbacctin (**13**, 10-DAB), which can be easily extracted in high yield from the leaves of the English yew tree *T. baccata* L. Taxotere was discovered by Frenchman Pierre Potier by making a minor modification of Taxol (replacing the benzoyl group on Taxol with a *tert*-butoxyl-carbonyl group).[11,12] Taxotere (**14**), about 1.5-fold more potent than Taxol, had annual sales of $1.54 billion in 2003.

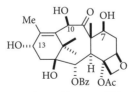

13, 10-deacetyl baccatin III (10-DAB)

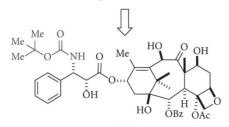

docetaxel (**14**, Taxotere)

The FDA approved Taxol for use in refractory ovarian cancer in December 1992, for breast cancer in 1994, and later for non–mall-cell lung cancer and Kaposi's sarcoma. By 2000, Taxol was the best-selling cancer drug of all time, with annual sales of $1.6 billion.

The raw material for isolating Taxol became an extremely contentious issue in the late 1980s and early 1990s. Since it takes one hundred years for a Pacific yew tree to become useful in terms of Taxol content, harvesting the trees for stem bark meant destruction of the forest. To make matters worse, the forest that harbors the trees is home to the endangered spotted owl. The battle raged for many years between the environmentalists, who wanted to save the trees, and cancer patients/oncologists, who were eager to get access to the drug. It ended abruptly in early 1993 when BMS started to use a semi-synthetic route to make Taxol which did not require the Pacific yew at all. Instead, BMS extracted 10-deacetylbacctin (13, 10-DAB) from *T. baccata*, the English yew, a common ornamental plant. BMS then used the side-chain installation process patented by Robert A. Holton at the Florida State University to make Taxol. More than three tons of English yew needles, a renewable source, need to be collected and processed in order to produce 1 kg of 10-DAB. The switch is worthwhile because Taxol cost $600,000 per kilogram at its most expensive, and costs nearly $400,000 per kilogram even now. The worldwide market for Taxol is about 400 kg per year. Currently, Taxol is produced in large fermentation tanks using plant cells.

■ 2 PHARMACOLOGY

2.1 Mechanism of Action

Many traditional anticancer drugs, such as cyclophosphamide (2, Cytoxan), 5-FU (3, fluorouracil) and methotrexate (4), work through, interact with, and cause irreparable damage to DNA; or to inhibit specific enzymes as exemplified by tamoxifen (5, Nolvadex) and raloxifene (6, Evista).

There is a third type of anticancer drug, known as antimitotics, whose MOA is through cell mitosis. One common characteristic of most cancer cells is their rapid rate of cell division. There are five stages of cell division: prophase, metaphase, anaphase, telophase, and interphase. Other cells are also adversely affected, but since cancer cells divide much faster than noncancerous cells, they are far more susceptible to antimitotic treatment. In order to accommodate antimitotics the cytoskeleton of a cell undergoes extensive restructuring. Microtubules become the scaffolding of the cell structure, forming the mitotic spindle, which is responsible for the segregation of chromosome during cell division. As the mitosis progresses, protein microtubules in the cell pull apart the chromosomes to each pole of the cell before cell division. Meanwhile, the cell walls begin to converge and the microtubules at the center of the convergence start to disassemble. The cell splits and the microtubules disappear in a process of depolymerization.

In the 1960s, colchicine (**15**) was found to be the first antimitotic. It works by binding to and inhibiting a protein called tubulin, the building block of microtubules. Colchicine–tubulin complex has been isolated and characterized. Tubulins come together to assemble microtubules in a process called polymerization, which leads to the arrest of cell division. Later on, the vinca alkaloids vinblastine (**16**, Velban) and vinorelbine (Navelbine) were discovered also to be antimitotics whose MOA is through inhibiting the polymerization of tubulin as well. Inhibition of microtubule formation arrests cell division at the metaphase stage of the cell cycle.

In 1977, Horwitz and Schiff began to elucidate the MOA of Taxol (**1**). Within a month, they were convinced that Taxol has a novel mechanism of action: Behaving like an antimitotic, it blocked cell division at the metaphase. But unlike colchicine (**15**) and vinblastine (**16**, Velban), which blocked cells in the mitotic phase of the cell cycle, cells treated with Taxol reorganized their microtubules so that distinct bundles of microtubules are formed in the cells.[9,13,14]

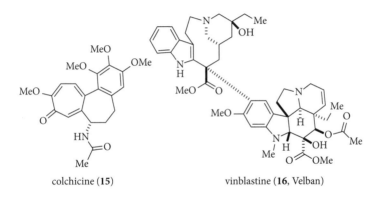

colchicine (**15**)   vinblastine (**16**, Velban)

In essence, Taxol hyperstabilizes the microtubule's structure. This destroys the cell's ability to use its cytoskeleton in a flexible manner. Specifically, Taxol binds to the β subunit of tubulin and the binding of Taxol locks these building blocks in place. The resulting Taxol–microtubule complex does not have the ability to disassemble. This adversely affects cell function because the shortening and lengthening of microtubules (termed dynamic instability) is necessary for their function as a mechanism to transport other cellular components. For example, during mitosis, microtubules position the chromosomes during their replication and subsequent separation into the two daughter-cell nuclei. In the presence of Taxol, cells can no longer divide into two daughter cells, and the tumor gradually dies. The ability of Taxol to polymerize tubulin into stable microtubules in the absence of any cofactors such as cold or $CaCl_2$ and to induce the formation of stable microtubules in cells is the unique characteristic of Taxol.[13]

Fig. 4.1 shows the Taxol binding site on mammalian β-tubulin of the Taxol–tubulin complex.[14] After considering data on Taxol binding to mammalian tubulin and recent modeling studies, it was hypothesized that differences in five key amino

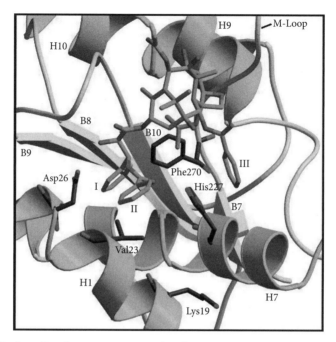

Fig. 4.1. Paclitaxel Binding Site on Mammalian β-Tubulin[14]

acids are responsible for the lack of Taxol binding to yeast tubulin. Mutagenesis experiment confirmed the hypothesis.

2.2 Structure–Activity Relationship

The SAR of naturally occurring taxane and baccatin III derivatives, converted to Taxol via attachment of the C-13 side chain was summarized by Georg and Potier.[15]

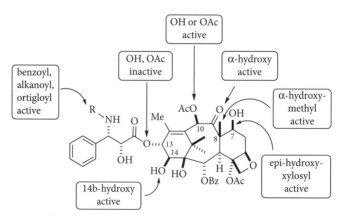

Fig. 4.2. SAR of Paclitaxel Analogs[15]

As shown in Fig. 4.2, the C-13 N-benzoyl-3′-phenylisoserine side chain is required for strong cytotoxic activity of taxane. It is worth noting that the N-benzoyl group of the C-13 side chain may be replaced by a tigloyl group such as cephlomannine without significant reduction in activity. Taxane with or without an acetyl group at the C-10-hydroxyl group has comparable activity. Epimerization at C-7 reduced activity slightly although replacing the C-7 hydroxyl group with a xylosyl substituent had better microtubule binding than the parent compound Taxol (**1**).

2.3 Bioavailability, Metabolism, and Toxicology

Just as remarkable as its novel MOA, Taxol is notorious for its low solubility. More than one researcher dubbed it a "sand-like" material. Indeed, Taxol's aqueous solubility is extremely low: approximately 6 μM (~5 mg/mL) although its solubility in organic solvents is better.[16] The target formulation concentration for intravenous infusion in humans was >5 mg/mL. Because it is highly insoluble in water, numerous formulations were investigated and the final product chosen by BMS was 30 mg of Taxol in 5 mL ampoules with 50% Cremophor EL and 50% anhydrous ethanol.[17] The concentration of Cremophor EL, known to cause histamine release (which could pose potential allergic reactions), is much higher than any other drug on the market. Before bolus injection, the content in the ampoule was diluted 5- to 20-fold with either 0.9% saline or 5% dextrose in water.

The pharmacokinetic data for Taxol vary significantly. Here the mean parameters are used by culling from the literature.[16] Upon IV administration, the concentration of Taxol in the blood decreases rapidly as drug distributes to the tissues with a mean distribution-phase half-life $T_{1/2\alpha}$ of 20.4 min. After the distribution phase is complete, an elimination phase appears; the mean terminal elimination half-life $T_{1/2\beta}$ is 2.9 h. Taxol's mean volume of distribution (V_{dss}) is 87 mL/m² (2.14 L/kg). Since the volume of distribution is larger than the total body water volume of 28.5 mL/m² (0.7 L/kg), it indicates that Taxol is distributed to a moderate degree to tissues and blood components.

As can be expected from the low solubility, Taxol binds rapidly and extensively to plasma protein, and a large fraction of the drug (>90–97%) is transported within the blood in the bound state. Little drug is excreted in the urine (<10%), and metabolites have been rarely detected in urine or blood. The principal mechanism for clearance of Taxol from the blood is hepatic metabolism. Clearance (Cl) can be expressed as the volume of plasma from which drug is removed per unit time. Taxol's mean Cl is 496 mL/min/m² with an area under the curve (AUC) of 3076 ng/mL•h.

Finally, C_{max}, the peak concentration of Taxol achieved during infusion, varies with the lengths of infusion. The C_{max} is higher for shorter infusion schedules (3–4 μM with a 6-h of infusion of 210–250 mg/m² of Taxol). The C_{max} is lower for longer infusion schedules (0.7–0.9 μM with a 24-h of infusion of 200 to 250 mg/m² of Taxol).[16,17]

In preclinical animal (rat, mouse, and rabbit) models[18] and human subjects,[19] the monohydroxylated Taxols are the major metabolites (Fig. 4.3). It was identified that CYP2C8, with a relatively high affinity and metabolic velocity, was largely responsible for oxidizing Taxol to its corresponding 6α-hydroxy-Taxol (**17**); whereas CYP3A4 was largely responsible for oxidizing Taxol to its corresponding 3′-p-hydroxy-Taxol (**18**). Both **17** and **18** may be further oxidized to 3π, 6α-dihydroxy-Taxol (**19**). Unlike those of Lipitor, Taxol's metabolites **17** and **18** are many-fold less active than Taxol and the dihydroxyl metabolite **19** is not active at all. The primary metabolite 6α-hydroxy-Taxol (**17**) has been isolated from bile, plasma, and feces.

The metabolic fate and disposition of Taxol in cancer patients has been determined using radiolabeled [3H]-Taxol.[20] Total urinary excretion was ~14.3% of the dose, with unchanged Taxol and an unknown polar metabolite as the main excretion products. Total fecal excretion was ~71.1%, with 6α-hydroxy-Taxol (**17**) being the largest component by far. Unchanged Taxol and four other metabolites could also be identified from fecal extracts. The plasma AUC for unchanged Taxol was ~20.5 μM h and that for total Taxol metabolites was 14.2 μM h. The half-life of total metabolites ~5.6 h, however, greatly exceeded that of unchanged Taxol (~2.9 h). Thus, at 5-h post-Taxol infusion, the plasma concentrations of the five metabolites together exceeded the Taxol concentration by 2.4-fold.

During the phase I single-agent trials using 150–250 mg/m^2 doses, the most threatening toxicity was the hypersensitivity reaction (HSR).[21] After some delay of the trials, the HSR was associated with the excipient used, Cremophor EL. Later it was found that a regimen of steroid and H1-histamine antagonist reduced the incidence of HSRs significantly. Another dose-limiting toxicity was a hematologic toxicity called myelo-suppression, specifically neutropenia. Later on, it was discovered during the phase II trials that a shorter infusion time (3 h vs. 24 h) greatly reduced Taxol's myelo-suppression effects.

Considering Taxol's MOA, it is not surprising that it is associated with neurotoxicity.[22] Microtubules play an important role in the development and maintenance of neurons. During development and regeneration, microtubule elongation contributes to the growth of neurites through interactions with the growth cone. In the mature neuron, microtubules are the major participating elements in mediating axonal transport and also provide important structural support for neurons. Therefore, it was not unexpected that neuronal development and function could be dramatically impaired by Taxol. The most common clinical neurotoxicity associated with Taxol administration has been a predominantly sensory distal neuropathy. It may be manifested as diminished sensation to pain, temperature, vibration, and/or proprioception.

As far as symptoms are concerned, Taxol's common side effects include nausea and vomiting, loss of appetite, change in taste, thinned or brittle hair, pain in the arm or leg joints lasting 2–3 days, changes in the color of the nails, and tingling in the hands or toes. More serious side effects such as unusual bruising or bleeding,

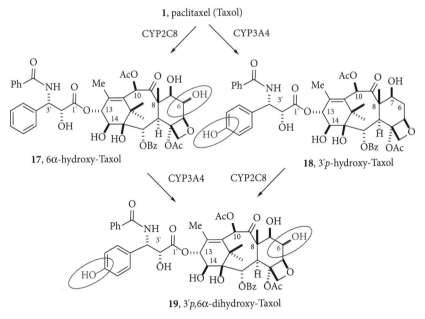

Fig. 4.3. Biotransformations of Paclitaxel

pain/redness/swelling at the injection site, change in normal bowel habits for more than 2 days, fever, chills, cough, sore throat, difficulty swallowing, dizziness, shortness of breath, severe exhaustion, skin rash, facial flushing, female infertility by ovarian damage, and chest pain can also occur.

■ 3 PROCESS SEMI-SYNTHESIS

In ae landmark paper in 1988,[23] a group of French chemists led by Andrew Greene revolutionized the landscape of Taxol field. Working with Potier, they achieved the semi-synthesis of Taxol from permanently accessible Taxol congener 10-deacetyl baccatin III (**13**, 10-DAB), which can be easily extracted in high yield from the leaves of English yew tree *T. baccata* L. While the yield of Taxol (**1**) from *dry* barks of Pacific yew tree *T. brevifolia* was merely 0.14 g/kg; the yield of 10-deacetyl baccatin III (**13**) was 1 g/kg of *fresh* leaves of the English yew. More importantly, through prudent harvesting, large amounts of **13** can be continually supplied with negligible effect on the yew population. In Greene's synthesis, as shown below, they selectively protected the C-7 alcohol as the corresponding TES ether, 7-O-TES-10-DAB (**20**), in 84–86% yield without significant silylation of the C-13 and C-15 hydroxyl groups. Subsequently, another selective hydroxyl group protection of the C-10 alcohol on **20** was achieved using 5 equiv of acetyl chloride to afford 7-O-TES-bacctin-III (**21**) in 84% yield. 7-O-TES-bacctin-III (**21**) would serve as the common intermediate for their and many others' key building block to make

Taxol (**1**), taxotere (**14**), and their analogs. Installation of the side chain was then accomplished by coupling **21** with readily available optically pure (2R,3S)-N-benzoyl-O-(1-ethoxyethyl)-3-phenyl-isoserine (**22**) using di-2-pyridyl carbonate (DPC) to produce ester **23**. Concomitant removal of the carefully chosen protecting groups at C-2′ and C-7 then delivered Taxol (**1**) in 89% yield.

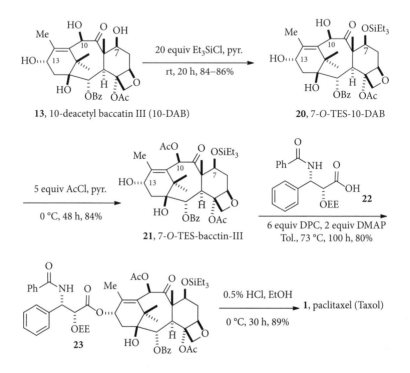

Greene's work laid the foundation for another breakthrough in Taxol synthesis. Robert Holton at Florida State University developed a semi-total synthesis using the metal alkoxides of **21** to open β-lactam ring **24** as the isoserine side chain.[24,25] The key operation entails deprotonation of alcohol **21** using n-BuLi, LDA, or other bases. Treatment of alkoxide of **21** with silyl-protected β-lactam ring **24** then gave the adduct, which was carefully deprotected using HF in pyridine. The overall yield for the two operations is greater than 80%. This strategy was later adopted and improved by BMS Process Chemistry, and it eventually became the manufacturing route.

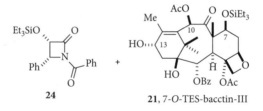

24

21, 7-O-TES-bacctin-III

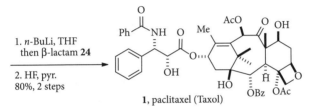

In Holton's initial patent, β-lactam **24** was prepared as a racemate. As shown below, benzaldehyde was converted to (*E*)-*N*-benzylidene-1,1,1-trimethylsilanamine (**25**). Meanwhile, ethyl 2-(triethyl-silyloxy)acetate was converted to ketene-like enolate using LDA. The "enolate" was coupled with **25** to form β-lactam **26**. Protection of β-lactam **26** with benzoyl chloride then furnished the key intermediate **24**. Of course, the synthesis of β-lactam **24** shown here is in the racemate form. One of Holton's enantiomerically selective syntheses of the β-lactam using a chiral oxazolidinone chiral auxiliary was published in 1993.[26]

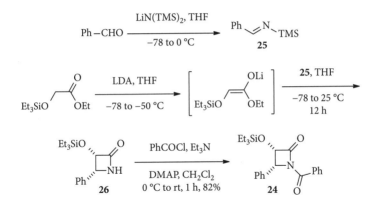

In 2001, a US patent was granted to BMS for a novel route of process for making Taxol.[27] Extensive experimentation showed that deprotonation of **27** using lithium *t*-buoxide as the base and DMF as the solvent at low temperature gave the cleanest C-7 alkoxide **28**. It was then treated with various electrophiles to give C-7 protected intermediate **29** as Boc, Cbz, Ac, etc. Esterification of **29** with (4*S*,5*R*)-2,4-diphenyl-4,5-dihydrooxazole-5-carboxylic acid (**30**) provided ester **31**, which was transformed to Taxol (**1**) in three additional steps.

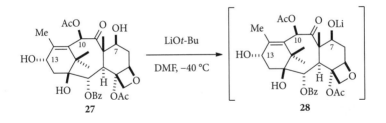

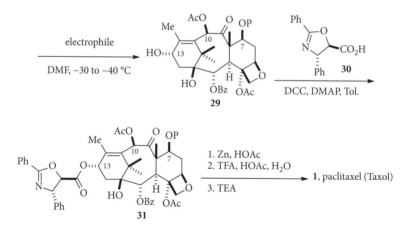

An alternative synthesis was also disclosed in the same patent.[27] Similar to Holton's approach, intermediate **29** was deprotonated with a base (lithium t-buoxide) to afford the C-13 alkoxide. Different from Holton's approach, the alkoxide was treated with β-lactam **31** with a 1-methyl-1-methoxyethyl ether protection instead of the TES protection. Presumably these changes would facilitate large-scale manufacturing in terms of ease of operations. Treatment of the resulting ester with TFA in acetic acid offered the C-7 protected Taxol **32**. Finally, removal of the protective group then delivered Taxol (**1**).

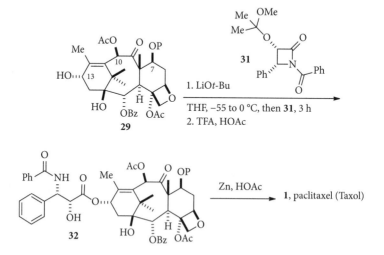

■ **4 TOTAL SYNTHESIS**

Six total syntheses of Taxol (**1**) have been accomplished thus far. A summary of their strategies is given here.[28]

4.1 Holton's Synthesis

Using (–)-camphor (**33**) or (–)-borneol as the starting material, tricyclic (–)-TES-β-patchoulol (**34**) may be prepared via the intermediacy of patchoulene oxide.[29,30] Epoxidation of **34** was followed by an epoxy-alcohol (**35**) fragmentation to afford bicyclic intermediate **36**, which was manipulated in a linear fashion to assemble **37** as the C-7 protected bacctin III. The alkoxide of **37** was generated using LiHMDS and it was quenched by β-lactam **24** to deliver Taxol after two deprotection steps.

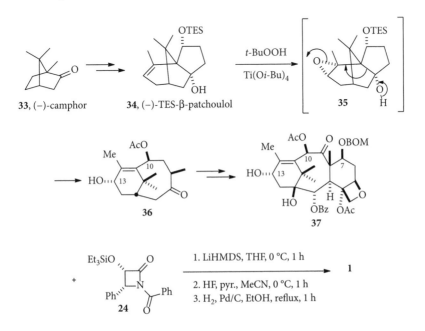

Holton's linear synthesis has an overall yield of 4–5% for total 38 chemical steps from (–)-TES-β-patchoulol (**34**), which requires an additional 18 steps from camphor.

4.2 Nicolaou's Synthesis

Nicolaou's synthesis is more convergent.[31] A Shapiro reaction between aryl hydrazone **38** and aldehyde **39** (whose preparation involved an elegant regioselective Diels–Alder reaction of a hydroxy α,β-unsaturated ester and a hydroxy-pyrone tethered with phenylboronic acid) assembled the adduct alcohol **40** as a single diastereomer in 82% yield. After five steps of functional group manipulations, the key intermediate was set as di-aldehyde **41**. The pivotal cyclization of **41** was achieved using a McMurry-type pinacol reaction established the taxoid ABC ring system as diol **42** in 23% yield. At this point, **42** was prepared as a racemate, which was resolved using (1S)-(–)-camphanic chloride and isolated the desired diastereomer using a standard column. Additional manipulations then provided appropriately decorated ABC ring as **20**, which was converted to Taxol (**1**) by coupling of the alkoxide of **20** generated by NaHMDS with β-lactam **24** to deliver Taxol after two deprotection steps.

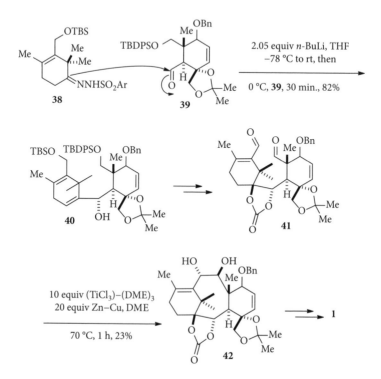

Nicolaou's convergent approach required approximately 34 steps. The key transformation of **41→42** using the McMurry pinacol coupling suffered a low yield of 23%, which is a testimony to the herculean efforts that Nicolaou and his co-workers made to accomplish the feat of the total synthesis of Taxol.

4.3 Danishefsky's Synthesis

Two years after Holton's and Nicolaou's total syntheses of Taxol were published, Danishefsky's group disclosed their version.[32] Their synthesis used the (+)-enantiomer of the Wieland–Miescher ketone (**44**) as his starting material. They obtained **44** in quantity by L-proline-induced aldolization of the prochiral trione **43**. The (+)-Wieland–Miescher ketone (**44**) was converted (in 25 steps!) to aldehyde **45**, reminiscent of Nicolaou's aldehyde **39**. Coupling of aldehyde **45**, with vinyl lithium **46** gave rise to adduct **47**. Eight Additional steps of functional group transformations of **47** provided the key intermediate **48**, which underwent an intramolecular Heck reaction to produce the taxoid ABC ring system **49** in 50% yield. Further 14 manipulations of **49** including installation of the isoserine side-chain then delivered Taxol.

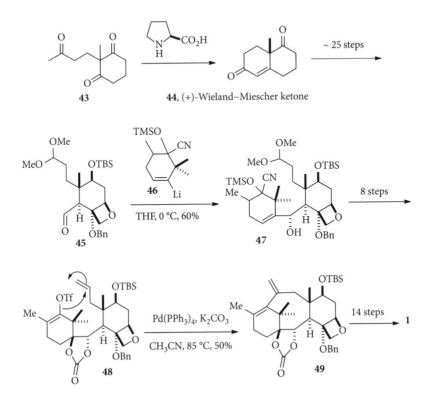

Danishefsky carried the CD ring system with the oxetane's functionality incorporated throughout the whole scheme, an audacious feat. Similar to that of Nicolaou's, it is convergent. Although it took about 48 steps, Danishefsky declared:[32] "Our synthesis, though arduous, involves no relays, no resolutions, and no recourse to awkwardly available antipode of the 'chiral pool'." His reference to "no resolutions" took a swipe at Nicolaou's maneuver. His comments on "antipode" are probably referred to Holton's synthesis, which was the antipode of the natural Taxol.

4.4 Wender's Synthesis

Wender's synthesis used pinene (**50**) as his starting material, which underwent air oxidation to give verbenone (**51**).[33,34] Six additional steps converted **51** to the key tricyclic intermediate **52** with the key operations involving a photochemical rearrangement of an enone to the chrysathernone skeleton and a Michael addition of a methyl cuprate to the propionate. Epoxidation of **52** selectively on the less sterically hindered, tri-substituted olefin produced the *syn* epoxy–alcohol **53**, which, upon treatment with DABCO, underwent a rearrangement to afford the AB ring system of Taxol as **54**. Later on, the C-ring was assembled using an aldol ring-closure. In all, it took 30 additional steps to transform the AB ring system **54** to baccatin III **55**. Using the Holton–Ojima protocol then delivered Taxol in the correct enantiomeric form. The total synthesis, involving 37 steps from verbenone (**51**), is the shortest and is viewed by some as the most elegant.

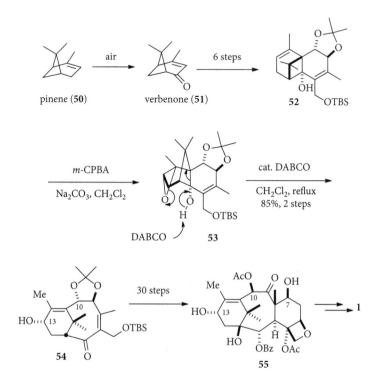

■ 5 CONCLUDING REMARKS

Taxol has made tremendous contributions to cancer therapy. Its exclusivity having expired in 2000, the generic form Taxol is now widely available. In addition to its contribution to helping cancer patients, Taxol also provided an opportunity for elucidation of its novel MOA, namely tubulin polymerization. The discovery also fueled interest in finding additional agents to work through the tubulin polymerization. Epothilones turned out to be a new class of tubulin polymerization agents.[35] Epothilone B (**56**) was first isolated in 1991. In 1997, it was demonstrated that epothilones are microtubule stabilization agents that maintain their cytotoxic effects against tumor cell lines that are resistant to Taxol. Chemists at BMS converted the lactone on epothilone B (**56**) to its corresponding lactam in an effort to boost its bioavailability. The resulting lactam, also known as azaepothilone, was

BMS-247550, which eventually was granted ixabepilone (**57**) as its USAN generic name. In 2007, the FDA approved ixabepilone (**57**, trade name Ixempra) for the treatment of advanced breast cancer, especially for Taxol-refractory patients.

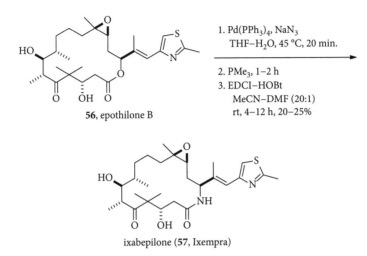

56, epothilone B

1. Pd(PPh$_3$)$_4$, NaN$_3$
   THF–H$_2$O, 45 °C, 20 min.

2. PMe$_3$, 1–2 h
3. EDCI–HOBt
   MeCN–DMF (20:1)
   rt, 4–12 h, 20–25%

ixabepilone (**57**, Ixempra)

■ 6 REFERENCES

1. Gaines, A.; Whiting, J. *Robert A. Winsberg and the Search for the Cause of Cancer,* Mitchell Lane Publishers: Bear, DE, 2001.

2. Weinberg. R. A. *Racing to the Beginning of the Road, The Search for the Origin of Cancer,* W. H. Freeman and Company: New York, 1998.

3. Varmus, H.; Weinberg, R. A. *Genes and Biology of Cancer,* Scientific American Library: New York, 1993.

4. Avendano, C.; Menendez, J. C. *Medicinal Chemistry of Anticancer Drugs,* Elsevier Science: Amsterdam, The Netherlands, 2008.

5. Piñeiro-Núñez, M. Raloxifene, Evista: a selective estrogen receptor modulator (SERM), in *Modern Drug Synthesis;* Li, J. J.; Johnson, D. S., Eds., Wiley: Hoboken, NJ, 2010, pp. 309–327.

6. Li, J. J. Aromatase inhibitors for breast cancer: exemestane (Aromasin), anastrozole (Arimidex) and letrozole (Femara), in *The Art of Drug Synthesis;* Li, J. J.; Johnson, D. S., Eds., Wiley: Hoboken, NJ, 2007, pp. 31–38.

7. Goodman, J.; Walsh, V. *The Story of Taxol: Nature and Politics in the Pursuit of an Anti-Cancer Drug,* Cambridge University Press: Oxford, 2001.

8. Oberlies, N., H.; Kroll, D. J. *J. Nat. Prod.* **2004**, *67*, 129–135.

9. Howitz, S. B. *J. Nat. Prod.* **2004**, *67,* 136–138.

10. Kingston, David G. I. *Chem. Commun.* **2001**, 867–880.

11. Guenard, D.; Gueritte-Voegelein, F.; Potier, P. *Acc. Chem. Res.* **1993**, *26*, 160–167.

12. Denis, J.-N.; Greene, A. E.; Guenard, D.; Gueritte-Voegelein, F.; Mangatal, L.; Potier, P. *J. Am. Chem. Soc.* **1988**, *110*, 5917–5919.

13. Howitz, S. B. *Trends Pharmacol. Sci.* **1992**, *13*, 134–136.

14. Gupta, M. L., Jr.; Bode, C. J.; Georg, G. I.; Himes, R. H. *PNAS* **2003**, *100*, 6394–6397.

15. (a) Georg, G. I.; Boge, T. C.; Cheruvallath, Z. et al. The medicinal chemistry of Taxol, in *Taxol: Science and Applications*, Suffness, M., Ed., CRC: Boca Raton, FL, 1995, pp. 317–375. (b) Guenard, D.; Gueritte-Voegelein, F.; Potier, P. *Acc. Chem. Res.* **1993**, *26*, 160–167.

16. Straubinger, R. M. Biopharmaceutics of paclitaxel (Taxol): formulation, activity, and pharmaco-kinetics *Taxol: Science and Applications*, Suffness, M., Ed., CRC: Boca Raton, FL, 1995, pp. 237–258.

17. Suffness, M. *Annu. Rep. Med. Chem.* **1993**, *28*, 305–314.

18. Sparreboom, A.; van Tellingen, O.; Nooijen, W. J.; Beijnen, J. H. *Anticancer Drugs* **1998**, *9*, 1–17.

19. Rochat, B. Role of Cytochrome P450 *Clin. Pharmacokinet.* **2005**, *44*, 349–366.

20. Walle, T.; Walle, U. K.; Kumar, G. N.; Bhalla, K. N. *Drug Metab. Dispos.* **1995**, *23*, 506–512.

21. Donehower, R. C.; Rowinsky, E. K. *Cancer Treat. Rev.* **1993**, *19(Suppl. C)*, 63–78.

22. Apfel, S. C. *Cancer Invest.* **2000**, *18*, 564–573.

23. Denis, J.-N.; Greene, A. E.; Guénard, L.; Guéritte-Voegelein, F.; Mangatal, l.; Potier, P. A *J. Am. Chem. Soc.* **1988**, *110*, 5917–5919.

24. Holton, R. A. *Metal Alkoxides*. U.S. Pat. 5, 274, 124, December 28, 1993.

25. Holton, R. A.; Biediger, R. J.; Boatman, P. D. Semisynthesis of Taxol and Taxotere, in *Paclitaxel: Science and Applications*, Suffness, M., Ed., CRC: Boca Raton, FL, 1995, pp. 97–119.

26. Holton, R. A.; Liu, J. H. *Bioorg. Med. Chem. Lett.* **1993**, *3*, 2475–2478.

27. Hudlický, T.; Reed, J. W. *The Way of Synthesis: Evolution of Design and Methods for Natural Products*, Wiley-VCH: Weinheim, Germany, 2007, pp. 499–524.

28. Gibson; F. S. *Synthesis of Taxol from Baccatin III By Protection of the 7-Hydroxyl of Baccatin III Using a Strong Base and an Electrophile*. U.S. Pat. 6,307,071, October 23, 2001.

29. Holton, R. A.; Somoza, C.; Kim, H. B. et al. *J. Am. Chem. Soc.* **1994**, *116*, 1597–1598.

30. Holton, R. A.; Kim, H. B.; Somoza, C. et al. *J. Am. Chem. Soc.* **1994**, *116*, 1599–1600.

31. Nicolaou, K. C.; Yang, Z.; Liu, J. J. et al. *Nature* **1994**, *6464*, 630–634.

32. Danishefsky, S. J.; Masters, J. J.; Young, W. B. et al. *J. Am. Chem. Soc.* **1996**, *118*, 2843–2859.

33. Wender, P. A.; Badham, N. F.; Conway, S. P. et al. *J. Am. Chem. Soc.* **1997**, *119*, 2755–2756.

34. Wender, P. A.; Badham, N. F.; Conway, S. P. *J. Am. Chem. Soc.* **1997**, *119*, 2757–2758.

35. Morihira, K.; Hara, R.; Kawahara, S. et al. *J. Am. Chem. Soc.* **1998**, *120*, 12980–12981.

36. Kusama, H.; Hara, R.; Kawahara, S et al. *J. Am. Chem. Soc.* **2000**, *122*, 3811–3820.

37. Mukaiyama, T.; Shiina, I.; Iwadare, H *Chem. Eur. J.* **1999**, *5*, 121–161.

38. Borzilleri, R. M.; Vite, G. D. *Drugs Fut.* **2002**, *27*, 1149–1163.

5   Imatinib Mesylate (Gleevec)

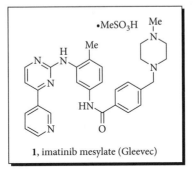

1, imatinib mesylate (Gleevec)

USAN:	*Imatinib Mesylate*
Brand Name:	*Gleevec (Novartis)*
Molecular Weight:	*589.71 (Parent, 493.60)*
FDA Approval:	*2001*
Drug Class:	*Protein-tyrosine Kinase Inhibitor*
Indications:	*Treatment of Chronic Myeloid Leukemia (CML) and Gastrointestinal Stromal Tumors (GIST)*
Mechanism of Action:	*Inhibiting a Set of More Than 8 Protein-Tyrosine Kinases*

Imatinib mesylate (**1**, Gleevec) is a protein-tyrosine kinase inhibitor for the treatment of chronic myeloid leukemia (CML) and gastrointestinal stromal tumors (GIST). It is the first orally bioavailable anticancer drug that only targets enzymes (protein kinases) that are specific to tumor cell growth but not required by healthy cells. Therefore, protein kinase inhibitors are also known as targeted cancer drugs or smart drugs.

Gleevec was Novartis's top performer in 2012 with sales of $4.6 billion.

■ 1 HISTORY

1.1 A Brief History of Cancer Drugs

Great strides had been made in the war against cancer with chemotherapy even before the emergence of protein kinase inhibitors.[1] For instance, prior to vinblastine (**1**, Velban) became available in 1964 for the treatment of lymphoma, the diagnosis of Hodgkin's disease (a cancer of the lymph nodes) was virtually a death sentence. Today there is a 90% chance of survival with the treatment by vinca

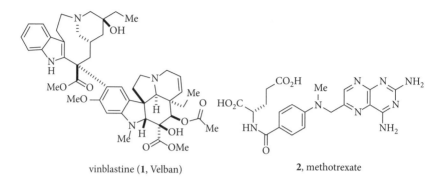

vinblastine (**1**, Velban)   **2**, methotrexate

alkaloids such as **1** and other chemotherapies. Similarly, when Sidney Farber discovered the effects of methotrexate (**2**, Trexall) on leukemia, it marked the beginning of the triumph over childhood leukemia.

Following Barnett Rosenberg's discovery of cisplatin (**3**, Platinol)'s effects on tumor cells in 1967, cisplatin and its analogs such as carboplatin (**4**, Paraplatin) and oxaliplatin (**5**, Eloxatin) contributed significantly in boosting the survival rate of patients with metastatic testicular cancer, ovarian tumors, and bladder cancer. Most significantly, breast cancer, a malady striking one in eight women, has been effectively managed via a plethora of treatments including surgery, radiation, and chemotherapies. The arsenal of chemotherapeutics for treating breast cancer includes SERMs such as tamoxifen (**6**) and raloxifene (**7**, Evista). Type I, II, and III aromatase inhibitors have now also been widely prescribed to combat breast cancers (more details may be found in chap. 4). Today, breast cancer is sometimes viewed as a chronic disease that can be managed, rather than a lethal disease.

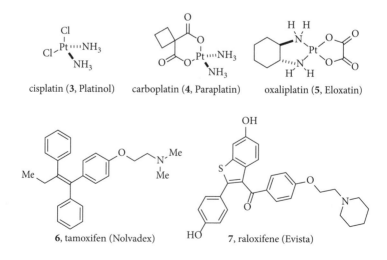

cisplatin (**3**, Platinol)   carboplatin (**4**, Paraplatin)   oxaliplatin (**5**, Eloxatin)

6, tamoxifen (Nolvadex)   **7**, raloxifene (Evista)

Despite the efficacy of the aforementioned chemotherapeutics, they kill cancer cells and normal cells with equal ferocity. (Some have compared chemotherapy to a "carpet bombing" strategy.) However, the reason these chemotherapies are effective is that cancer cells divide at much faster rate than normal cells; therefore, chemotherapies kill more malignant cells than healthy cells.

Chemotherapies invariably come with significant side effects rooted. For example, hair follicle cells have a physiologically high mitosis rate; therefore, chemotherapies kill them faster than other healthy cells. In the same vein, other common side effects of chemotherapy include diarrhea (because ephithelial renewal is inhibited), bone marrow suppression (because granulopoiesis, thrombopoiesis, cytopoiesis, and erythropoiesis are inhibited), and lymph node damage (because of lymphocyte multiplication inhibition causes immune weakness). These toxicities manifest as damage to the gastrointestinal tract, bone marrow, nervous system, kidneys, heart, or pancreas. Therefore, a cancer treatment that kills the cancer cells while leaving the healthy cells alone is highly desirable. In other words, a strategy with the same or better efficacy as chemotherapy but without its toxicities is needed.

Protein kinase inhibitors fit the bill. In contrast to the "carpet bombing" strategy of chemotherapy, protein kinase inhibitors are akin to "precision bombs" that only kill cancer cells, and are thus devoid many of the toxicities (and therefore the side effects) that plagued conventional chemotherapies.

1.2 Treatments of Chronic Myeloid Leukemia

Among the many subtypes of leukemia, a rare but particularly ferocious form is chronic myeloid leukemia (CML) where "myeloid" indicates that it is marrow-related. CML is a hematologic stem cell disorder caused by an acquired abnormality in the DNA of the stem cells in bone marrow and is characterized by abnormally high white blood cell counts.[2] CML is one of the four main types of leukemia, striking about 5,000,000 patients a year in the US. It mainly affects adults between the ages of 50 and 60.

CML was first described by Rudolf Virchow, among others, around 1845. In 1872, Ernst Neumann observed that CML cells originated in the bone marrow. One of the early treatment options for treating CML was a bone marrow transplant. However, not only was a matching donor needed, but the procedure was highly risky with a survival rate of only 50%. Effective control of blood counts became feasible in 1959 with the orally bioavailable alkylating agent busulfan (**8**, butane-1,4-bis-mesylate) synthesized by Geoffrey Timmis at Burrroughs Wellcome. Busulfan acts on primitive stem cells and is rarely used today because of its severe, toxic side effects. The better-tolerated hydroxyurea (**9**), developed by BMS and the University of Chicago, became available in 1969. A ribonucleotide reductase inhibitor, hydroxyurea (**9**) became a commonly used cytotoxic agent in the treatment of CML thanks to both the fast onset of its effect and relatively low toxicities. Soon afterward, interferon-α was found to induce durable major cytogenetic responses (decreasing the number of Philadelphia chromosome cells) and long-term survival, although in only a small fraction of patients, reducing the white cell count to tolerable levels. It became for a while the most popular treatment for CML. Unfortunately, in addition to being a biologic that has to be given intravenously, the flu-like side effect brought on by interferon makes it less desirable. Another intravenous drug, cysteine arabinose (**10**, Ara-C, cytarabine), came along later. Finally, cortisone (**11**) and prednisone (**12**) at high doses are also known to kill leukemic lymphocytes and lymphoblasts.

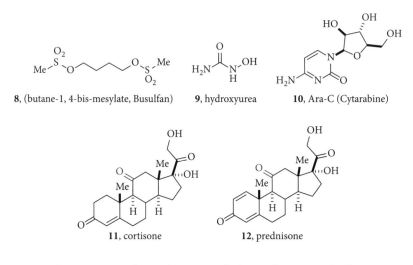

8, (butane-1, 4-bis-mesylate, Busulfan)   **9**, hydroxyurea   **10**, Ara-C (Cytarabine)

11, cortisone   **12**, prednisone

Again, drugs **8–12** and interferon are all chemotherapy, and all possess significant toxicities. Conversely, Novartis's Gleevec (**1**) specifically targets a protein kinase Abl (short for "Abelson; see below) for the treatment of CML. Gleevec (**1**) is the first marketed drug whose MOA is via inhibition of a protein kinase, functioning as a signal transduction inhibitor (STI). Imatinib represents a new paradigm in cancer therapy, revolutionizing the treatment of CML and GIST patients as an oral drug with side effects that are both relatively fewer and more tolerable than those of hydroxyurea (**9**), Ara-C (**10**), and interferon.

In 1960, Philadelphia cytogeneticists Peter Nowel and David Hungerford described an abnormally small G-group chromosome that we now call the Philadelphia chromosome (Ph) in CML patients. This was a seminal discovery as it unequivocally proved that CML cancer was directly linked to an abnormality of DNA.

In 1970, Herbert Abelson, working with David Baltimore, isolated a transforming gene from a specific variant of the Moloney leukemia virus. In 1973, Janet Rowley recognized that Ph was the product of a reciprocal translocation between chromosomes 9 and 22. In the 1980s, the human Abelson gene (Abl) was found on human chromosome 9 but translocated to the Ph chromosome in CML. Also in the 1980s, the translocation partners were identified as breakpoint cluster region (Bcr) and Abl, followed by the discovery that unregulated tyrosine kinase activity is critical to Bcr–Abl's ability to transform cells. The disappearance of the Ph chromosome in CML patients who underwent allotransplants, the first cures of CML, was also reported.

In 1986 and 1987, David Baltimore and his postdoctoral fellow, Owen Witte, published two articles in *Science* identifying Bcr–Abl as a tyrosine kinase. Like epidermal growth factor receptor (EGFR), Bcr–Abl is an enzyme that carries out signal transduction through the transfer of phosphate groups to specific amino acids (tyrosine in this case) on a protein. As a consequence, the cells receiving the signal begin dividing uncontrollably, thus triggering cell proliferation and leukemia. The hallmark of CML is the expression of Bcr–Abl. In effect, Baltimore and Witte identified the Bcr–Abl gene as the cause of CML. It then made sense that blocking the Bcr–Abl enzyme and stopping the faulty signal transduction would stave off the production of white blood cells. CML is one of very few cancers that has been directly linked to a *single* oncogene (i.e., Bcr–Abl). Most cancers are associated with at least two, and often more, oncogenes. In 1990, a faithful murine disease model for CML was established, which greatly boosted the research in the field. In 1992, Alexander Levitzki from Israel proposed the use of Abl inhibitors to treat leukemia driven by Abl oncogenes. In reality, at that time many hurdles still existed on the road to an oral drug for combating CML.

1.3 Protein Kinase Inhibitors

In 1966 Fischer and Krebs published their seminal work on protein phosphorylation (i.e., adding a phosphate) and its regulatory function in cellular pathways.[3] As shown in Fig. 5.1, protein kinases modulate intracellular signal transduction by catalyzing the phosphorylation of specific proteins. For example, protein phosphorylation catalyzed by protein kinase C (PKC) is activated by diacylglycerol (DAG). On the contrary, protein *phosphatases* function through *de*-phosphorylation of proteins to modulate biological activities, while concomitantly ATP (adenosine triphosphate, **13**) loses one molecule of phosphate to give ADP (adenosine diphosphate, **14**). Many cellular processes are the result of the interplay between phosphorylation by protein kinases and dephosphorylation by protein phosphatases.

Protein kinases comprise more than 518 members of ATP-regulated cellular or membrane-bound proteins that are capable of donating phosphate groups to target proteins.[4] They regulate critical cellular processes including gene transcription and cell growth, proliferation, and differentiation, often through complex and interactive processes. Since protein kinases are responsible for signal transduction, turning on and off the switches for cancer cells to grow, they are strongly implicated in cancer. Oncogenic kinases[5,6] are known to cause aberrant and often uncontrollable cellular phosphorylation and lead to tumor formation. By blocking the functions of protein kinases, it may be possible to stop cancer growth. Therefore kinase inhibitors hold great potential as anticancer therapeutics.

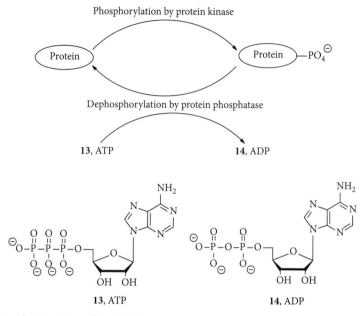

Fig. 5.1. The Functions of Protein Kinase

Protein kinases can be classified according to the amino acid residue that is phosphorylated in the cellular process. Consequently, there are tyrosine-specific kinases and serine/threonine kinases. Tyrosine kinases are a family of tightly regulated enzymes involved in phosphorylation to tyrosine, and the aberrant activation of various members of this family is one of the hallmarks of cancer. Tyrosine phosphorylation has been linked to multiple cell growth and differentiation pathways. Therefore, protein kinase inhibition is an area for therapeutic intervention against a variety of diseases such as cancer, inflammatory disorders, and diabetes.

Because protein kinases are selective against cancer cells, it is hoped that protein kinase inhibitors will have good efficacy without the toxicities associated with older chemotherapies. They promise a kinder, gentler, and more effective method for cancer treatment. Hence, protein kinase inhibitors are called *targeted cancer drugs*.

As a testimony to the importance of the protein kinase field, Bishop and Varmus received the 1989 Nobel Prize (for Physiology or Medicine) for their work on oncogenic kinases.[7] In 2001, Nurse and Hunt, along with Hartwell, were also awarded the Nobel Prize for their work in elucidating the role of cyclins and cyclin-dependent kinases (CDK) in regulating cell cycles.[8]

Biologics as protein kinase inhibitors were the first approved cancer treatments by inhibiting kinases. The first three are trastuzumab (Herceptin), cetuximab (Erbitux), and bevacizumab (Avastin). As of 2014, more than 12 monoclonal antibodies (mAbs) have been approved by the FDA for the treatments of cancers.

Genentech's Herceptin is a bioengineered *humanized* monoclonal antibody (shown in Fig. 5.2) for treating breast cancer. It was the first targeted cancer drug. Herceptin inhibits a human cellular oncogene—epidermal growth-factor receptor-2 (EGFR-2), also known as the HER-2/neu gene. Trastuzumab (Herceptin) was 95%t human and 5% murine (it is known as a chimeric antibody). It was approved by the FDA for treatment of HER-2 over-expressed metastatic breast cancers in 1998.[9]

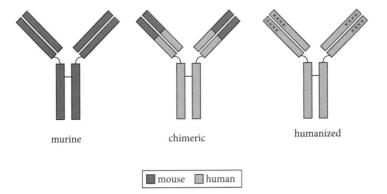

murine   chimeric   humanized

■ mouse □ human

Fig. 5.2. From Murine to Humanized mAb

Cetuximab (Erbitux) is a chimeric monoclonal antibody of EGF receptors, which are found in a third of solid cancer tumors. It was approved by the FDA for clinical use in 2004 to treat EGFR-expressing metastatic colorectal cancer.[10] Genentech's Avastin vindicated the anti-angiogenesis approach to fighting cancer. Avastin, a humanized monoclonal antibody against vascular endothelial cell growth factor (VEGF) receptor,[11] is the first drug to be marketed that works through the anti-angiogenesis mechanism.[12] It is 96% human and 4% murine.[13]

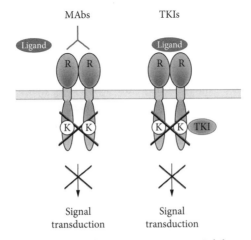

Fig. 5.3. Monoclonal antibodies (MAbs) vs. Tyrosine Kinase Inhibitors (TKIs)

The success of the aforementioned monoclonal antibodies in fighting cancers opened the floodgates to using small-molecule protein kinase inhibitors as oral drugs. Monoclonal antibodies left much to be desired since they are very expensive to make—manufactured by growing an enormous number of genetically identical ovary cells from hamsters in huge vats. In addition, because they are large proteins that do not survive in the gut they can only be administered by infusion. Oral drugs would, on the other hand, be cheaper to make and easier to swallow, so to speak.

So far, clinical studies have begun on hundreds of small-molecule kinase inhibitors. Most of these target the highly conserved ATP-binding site, leading to concerns about kinase selectivity. However, more than 20 small-molecule kinase inhibitors have overcome this early skepticism and have achieved regulatory approval as targeted antitumor therapeutics. As shown in Fig. 5.3, monoclonal antibodies bind to the receptors at the exterior of the cell's membrane whereas small molecule protein kinase inhibitors penetrate the cell's membrane and block the enzyme's function in the interior of the cell. Interestingly, most kinase inhibitors are flat aromatic compounds that mimic the adenine portion of ATP (13).

The first (in 2001) small-molecule kinase inhibitor on the market was Gleevec (1) for the treatment of CML and GIST. The second was AstraZeneca's gefitinib (Iressa, 15). An EGFR inhibitor, Iressa was launched in 2003 for the treatment of locally advanced or metastatic non–small-cell lung cancer. While Iressa's efficacy for Caucasian cancer patients saw mixed results, a subset analysis from a large clinical trial showed robust efficacy in patients of Asian origin with refractory advanced non–small-cell lung cancer.[14]

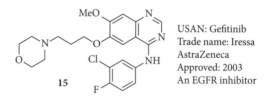

USAN: Gefitinib
Trade name: Iressa
AstraZeneca
Approved: 2003
An EGFR inhibitor

15

Sunitinib maleate (16, Sutent, SU11248) was discovered by Sugen, which later became part of Pfizer.[15] Sutent is an orally active drug that exhibits potent antiangiogenic activity through the inhibition of multiple receptor tyrosine kinases (RTKs). Specifically, 16 inhibits vascular EGFR, vascular endothelial growth factor receptor1 (VEGFR1), VEGFR2, and VEGFR3 and platelet-derived growth factor receptors-α (PDGFR-α) and PDGFR-β. In addition, Sutent also targets receptors implicated in tumerogenesis including fetal liver tyrosine kinase receptor 3 (Flt3) and stem-cell factor receptor (c-KIT). A drug with a multitarget profile is less likely to lead to drug resistance than a compound that displays selectivity for a single kinase. Furthermore, drugs that act on multiple pathways simultaneously may be more efficacious than single-target agents.

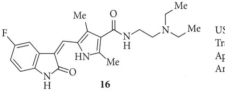

USAN: Sunitinib
Trade name: Sutent Pfizer
Approved: 2006
An angiogenesis inhibitor

16

Unfortunately, although the response rates for patients on first-line therapy with imatinib (**1**) are very high, approximately 22–41% of patients develop resistance to it—a significant percentage due to specific mutation in the Bcr–Abl kinase domain. Dasanitib (**17**, Sprycel), a dual Bcr–Abl and Src kinase inhibitor, is a good choice as a second-line tyrosine kinase inhibitor in Gleevec-resistant CML patients harboring Bcr–Abl kinase domain mutations.[16] It is likely that dasanitib (**17**) binds to different loops from those of Gleevec (**1**).

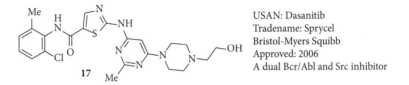

USAN: Dasanitib
Tradename: Sprycel
Bristol-Myers Squibb
Approved: 2006
A dual Bcr/Abl and Src inhibitor

17

Nilotinib (**18**, Tasigna), Novartis's follow-up to Gleevec (**1**), is an attempt to treat Gleevec-resistant CML patients.[17]

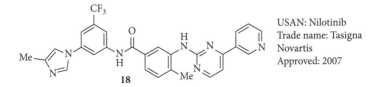

USAN: Nilotinib
Trade name: Tasigna
Novartis
Approved: 2007

18

In addition to **1** and **15–18**, there are about a dozen additional small-molecule protein kinase inhibitors that have been approved by the FDA for the treatment of cancer. They include axitinib (Inlyta, Pfizer, 2012), bosutinib (Bosulib, Pfizer, 2012), cabozantinib (Cometriq, Exelixis, 2012), cetuximab (Erbitux, ImClone, 2006), crizotinib (Xalkori, Pfizer, 2011), erlotinib (Tarceva, Genentech, 2005), lapatinib (Tykerb, GSK, 2007), pazopanib (Votrient, GSK, 2009), ponatinib (Iclusig, Ariad, 2012),[18] ruxolitinib (Jakafi, Incyte, 2011), sorafenib (Nexavar, Bayer, 2005),[19] vemurafenib (Zelboraf, Roche, 2011). Among these, bosutinib (Bosulib) is a promising candidate for third-line use in patients who fail on second-line TKI (tyrosine kinase inhibitor) therapy, and is being explored as a second-line therapy in its own right.

1.4 Genesis of Gleevec

In 1985, Alex Matter of Ciba-Geigy in Basel, Switzerland embarked on an ambitious oncology program targeting kinases. He and his colleague Nick Lydon did not make much progress until Brian Druker at Dana-Farber suggested that Ciba-Geigy work on targeting the Bcr–Abl kinase for CML in 1988. At the time it was already known that Bcr–Abl is an abnormal protein tyrosine kinase produced by the specific chromosomal abnormality called the Philadelphia chromosome and that this chromosome is a marker for CML. Two additional pieces of information aided their work: A few years earlier, Japanese scientists showed that staurosporine (**19**), an indole natural product, inhibited the receptor of PKC.[20] And, in 1988, Alexander Levitzki showed that selectivity could be achieved for EGFR. In a *Science* paper,[21] Levitzki revealed that a series of simple dicyanobenzylidenes such as **20** and carboxybenzylidenes could block EGF-dependent cell proliferation. The dicyanobenzylidenes were among the first selective small molecule EGFR kinase inhibitors.

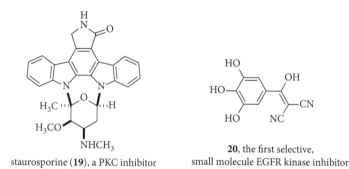

staurosporine (**19**), a PKC inhibitor

20, the first selective,
small molecule EGFR kinase inhibitor

There are more than 500 protein kinases, which all bear an uncanny structural resemblance to each other. To create a molecule that selectively targets Bcr–Abl required not only ingenuity, but also fantastic luck. An unselective inhibitor would have undesirable toxicity. In addition, since most protein kinase inhibitors resemble the adenosine molecule on ATP, they are mostly flat molecules and are notoriously insoluble; insoluble compounds cannot penetrate the cell membranes. The Bcr–Abl protein is located on the interior of cells, whereas the EGFR protein is extracellular, extruding out of the surface of cell membrane; thus it is more accessible. To bind to the Bcr–Abl protein, the drug has to penetrate the cell membrane or it will be completely useless.

Phenylaminopyrimidine **21** was initially identified by Ciba-Geigy from a high through-put screening (HTS) as a PKC-α inhibitor with an IC_{50} of approximately 1 μM. It did not inhibit Abl and PDGFR. Intensive SAR studies involving more than 300 analogs eventually led to STI571, which later became Gleevec (**1**) (Fig. 5.4). After STI571 was made, protein binding and later cellular assays by the biologists revealed that not only was it a potent blocker for the phosphorylation of

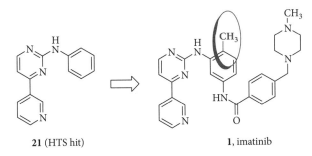

21 (HTS hit)   1, imatinib

Fig. 5.4. Evolution of the screening lead **21** to imatinib (**1**)

the Bcr–Abl kinase, it was also selective against most of the major kinases that they screened. In 1993, Druker also tested STI571 in protein and cellular models. He observed that STI571 killed CML cells without harming the healthy cells. STI571 subsequently showed sufficient efficacy in animal (murine) models.

In 1996, just when Novartis (Ciba-Geigy merged with Sandoz in March 1996 to become Novartis) was getting ready for the phase I clinical trials, a crushing piece of data came in: Severe liver toxicity was observed in both dogs and rats, which was a big blow to the project. However, Druker argued the disparity between dogs and humans is huge and results from a species closer to humans would be more relevant. Indeed, monkey toxicity studies revealed that STI571 had no significant liver toxicity at reasonable doses. Although the phase I clinical trial was not intended to gauge efficacy, those trials showed spectacular results. An added bonus was that the half-life of the drug in human was found to be 5 times longer than in animal models, allowing a once-daily regimen. STI571 arrested CML cells and left healthy cells alone.

Clinical trials initiated by Druker rapidly established STI571's activity in patients with CML. Novartis, encouraged by the unprecedented efficacy observed in phase I, took an unorthodox approach and moved the production to a fast-track status. The 12-step synthesis of STI571 in the manufacturing process was accomplished in an astonishingly short time—1.6 tons of STI571 were prepared in only 12 months, as opposed to the normal 24-month period.[22] Successful phase II trials in 1999 showed that the drug worked on all three phases of CML: chronic, accelerated, and blast. Novartis was able to submit a New Drug Application (NDA) in March 2001 armed with just the phase II results. For their part, the FDA approved it on May 10, 2001 in a record time of two and a half months. STI571 (imatinib, Gleevec) went through clinical trials faster and received approval as the first-line treatment of CML (and for the indication of GIST) from the FDA faster than any cancer therapy in history.

Gleevec revolutionized the treatment of CML as an oral drug with relatively few and more-tolerable side effects in comparison to hydroxyurea (**9**), Ara-C (**10**), and interferon. The remarkable clinical effectiveness of Gleevec validated the promise that targeted cancer therapy with a kinase inhibitor is possible. It has become a new paradigm in biomedical research.

■ 2 PHARMACOLOGY

2.1 Mechanism of Action

With Gleevec on the market, numerous studies to further understand the drug were undertaken. One study indicated that Gleevec actually blocks a panel of 8 protein kinases including Bcr–Abl, PDGFR kinase, c-Kit, and 5 others. The fact that Gleevec also inhibits another tyrosine kinase receptor, the c-Kit receptor that is associated with GIST, opened the door to use it to treat GIST.

Gleevec (**1**) is a tyrosine kinase inhibitor. An important characteristic of it is that it is an ATP-competitive inhibitor. It binds at the ATP binding site and blocks ATP binding thereby inhibiting kinase activities. Gleevec (**1**) exerts its pharmacological effect by first binding to a pocket of the Abl kinase domain.[23] Since the Bcr–Abl protein is located on the interior of cells, Gleevec (**1**) has to penetrate the cell membrane to bind to the Bcr–Abl protein.

The enzymatic in vitro test of Gleevec (**1**) against v-Abl-tyrosine kinase showed that it is a potent inhibitor with an IC_{50} = 38 nM. However, in cell, the IC_{50} is only 250 nM for the inhibition of the autophosphorylation of v-Abl. Nonetheless, what makes Gleevec an efficient drug is its excellent bioavailability (98% in humans), which allows for once daily oral treatment.

2.2 Structure–Activity Relationship

For the initial in vitro screen, the compounds were assayed for the inhibition of seven enzymes including four tyrosine kinases (v-Abl, PDGFR-kinase, EGFR-kinase, and c-Src) and three serine/threonine kinases (PKC_α, PKC_δ and PKA). The initial HTS hit **21** had an IC_{50} of 1.8 μM inhibiting the enzyme v-Abl kinase. While it was a weak inhibitor for PKC_α (IC_{50}, 10.5 μM) and PKC_δ (IC_{50}, 39 μM), respectively, **21** was completely inactive in inhibiting PDGFR-kinase, EGFR-kinase, c-Src, and PKA (Scheme 1).[24] Decoration of the phenylaniline moiety with various substituents did not result in impressive improvements in potency for v-Abl. For instance, compound **22** had an IC_{50} of 1.5 μM against v-Abl. However, more significantly, introduction of the "flag-methyl group" at the 6-position of the phenyl ring abolished the activity against PKC-α. That was a breakthrough because now they knew that they could make *selective* inhibitors against the v-Abl kinase!

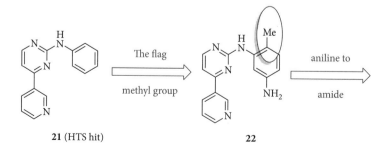

21 (HTS hit)   **22**

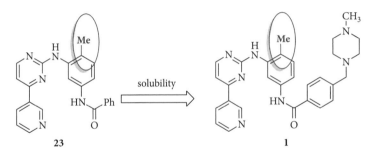

Scheme 1. Evolution from the screening lead **21** to imatinib (**1**)

With that knowledge in hand, the medicinal chemists installed amides using compound **22** as their template. The resulting amides increased the potency and selectivity. Take compound **23** as an example: It had an IC_{50} of 1.5 µM against v-Abl and was completely inactive against all other kinases tested except PDGFR (IC_{50}, 0.1 µM). This turned out to be a trend for this structure–activity relationship (SAR) and imatinib (**1**) itself has an IC_{50} of 0.0.5 µM against v-Abl. Ironically, this lack of selectivity against PDGFR might have made Gleevec a better drug.

In order to increase water solubility and thus bioavailability, Zimmermann installed a piperazine ring, which was later shown by X-ray crystallography to provide additional binding to the Bcr–Abl. Indeed, Gleevec (**1**) had an IC_{50} of 0.038 µM against v-Abl. It was synthesized in August 1992, a mere 2 years after Zimmerman began. Certainly he was a very good chemist, but luck probably played some role in this discovery because Ciba-Geigy made just around 300 compounds before Gleevec (**1**) was discovered!

A brief SAR table is shown in Table 5.1. When the fragments were closer to ideal, the impact of the "flag-methyl group" manifested in greater aptitude. For

TABLE 5.1. *SAR Table: The Enzymatic Profile IC_{50} (µM)*

Number	v-Abl-K	EGFR	c-Src	PDGFR	PKA	PKC_a	PKC_δ
21	1.8	100	>100	>10	>500	10.5	39
22	1.5	>100	>100	>10	>500	240	>500
23	0.4	65	>100	0.1	>500	72	>500
1	0.038	>100	>100	0.05	>500	>100	>100
24	0.1	>100	7.8	0.2	475	n.d.	n.d.

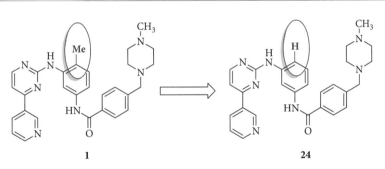

1   24

instance, simply abolishing the methyl group on **1** led to the resulting compound **24** having an IC_{50} of 0.1 μM against v-Abl—a nearly 3-fold drop in potency!

2.3 Bioavailability, Metabolism, and Toxicology

The bioavailability of Gleevec (**1**) is remarkably high (>97%).[25-28] It is highly soluble in water (200 mg/mL) and soluble in aqueous buffers at a pH of 5.5 or less. In vitro, it is strongly protein bound (95%), mainly to albumin and α1-acid glycoprotein.

After oral administration, Gleevec is absorbed rapidly in CML patients, with C_{max} reached at approximately 1–2 h postdose, and the compound is detected in plasma after 30 min. Following oral administration of ^{14}C-labeled Gleevec (**1**), the radioactivity in plasma suggests that more than 80% of the dose is absorbed.[25] The drug is extensively distributed into body tissue. The absolute bioavailability of Gleevec (**1**) is higher than 97% after oral administration of a single dose of 400 mg in the form of either four 100-mg capsules or an oral solution, compared with an intravenous (IV) infusion of 100 mg.[28]

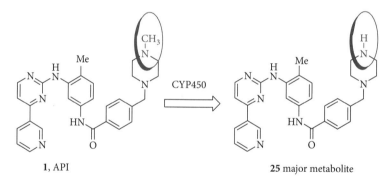

1, API   **25** major metabolite

Gleevec metabolism occurs in the liver and is mediated by CYP450, largely by the CYP3A4 subtype.[25,29-31] The major metabolite is the *N*-demethylation product **25**, also known as CGP74588. Metabolite **25** has in vitro potency similar to the parent drug, but its plasma AUC is only 16% of the AUC for the API **1**. Since CYP3A4 is the major enzyme responsible for Gleevec (**1**) metabolism, a patient on chronic phenytoin therapy (a CYP3A4 inducer) who received 350 mg of Gleevec (**1**) daily had an AUC_{0-24} about one-fifth of the typical Gleevec (**1**) AUC_{0-24}. When Gleevec (**1**) is co-administered with a single 400 mg dose of ketoconazole, a CYP3A4 inhibitor, AUC_{0-24} increases significantly. Furthermore, Gleevec (**1**) increased the mean C_{max} and AUC of simvastatin, a CYP3A4 substrate.

TABLE 5.2. *Pharmacokinetics parameters of imatinib mesylate (**1**)*

	C_{max} μg/L	T_{max} hr	$T_{1/2}$ hr	AUC_{0-24} μg*hr /L
Imatinib mesylate (**1**) 600 mg p. o.	3925	0.5–3.0	10–23	59535

Gleevec's AUC is dose proportional at the recommended daily dose range of 400–600 mg. Approximate 81% of the dose is eliminated within 7 days, 68% in feces and 13% in urine. The half-lives of Gleevec (**1**) and its main metabolite **25** are 18 and 40 h, respectively. Some key pharmacokinetics parameters of Gleevec (**1**) for humans are listed in Table 5.2.

As far as toxicology is concerned, the most common Gleevec (**1**) adverse events were nausea, vomiting, myalgia, edema, and diarrhea.[29] Elevated liver enzymes and/or bilirubin were reported in 2.6% of patients (27 out of 1,027 patients) in one clinical trial.

■ 3 SYNTHESIS

3.1 Discovery Synthesis

While both chemists, a medicinal (aka discovery) chemist has a completely different job description than a process chemist. A medicinal chemist would prefer to develop a "modular" synthetic methodology that would allow him/her to make a maximal number of analogs from a common intermediate. This is even more important these days when Contract Research Organizations (CRO) in China and India can make the intermediates on the cheap. On the other hand, the lead compound has already been selected when the process chemist gets involved. So his/her job is to optimize the route to synthesize this particular compound or a small class of compounds.

When Zimmermann and his colleagues were pursuing a lead compound for the Abl kinase, they took a synthetic approach that would yield as many and as diverse analogs as possible so they could explore the SAR as broadly as possible.

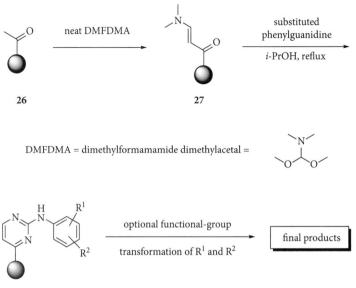

● = heterocycles or substituted phenyl

Scheme 2. The Discovery Route for Imatinib (**1**)

As shown in Scheme 2, ketone **26** was treated with dimethylformamamide dimethylacetal (DMFDMA) to afford enaminone **27**.[24] Subsequent treatment of **27** with substituted phenylguanidine with NaOH in refluxing *i*-PrOH then produced 2-phenylaminopyrimidine **28**. Additional functional group transformations then delivered the final product **29**.

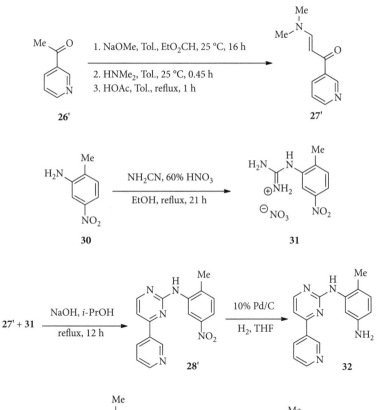

Scheme 3. The Discovery Route Specific for Imatinib (**1**)

Specifically for the synthesis of Gleevec (**1**), its discovery synthetic route was disclosed in two patents by Zimmermann.[32,33,34] As shown in Scheme 3, deprotonation of the methyl group on 3-acetylpyridine (**26′**) using freshly prepared sodium methoxide afforded an enolate. Condensation of the enolate with ethyl formate was followed by exchange with dimethylamine to produce 3-dimethylamino-1-(3-pyridyl)-2-propen-1-one (**27′**). Alternatively, **27′** could be prepared from the condensation of **26′** and N,N-dimethylformamide dimethylacetal (DMFDMA) as shown in Scheme 2.

Meanwhile, 2-amino-4-nitrotoluene (**30**), with the nitro group serving as a masked amine group, was prepared as a nitrate from nitration of 2-amino-toluene. Condensation of **30** with cyanamide and nitric acid in refluxing ethanol provided guanidinium nitrate **31**. It was purified by taking advantage of precipitation as a purification technique.

Subsequently, 2-phenylaminopyrimidine **28′** was assembled by treating enaminone **27′** and guanidinium nitrate **31** with NaOH in refluxing isopropanol. Similar to **27′**, **28′** was also precipitated from the respective reaction mixtures by the addition of insolubilizing solvents.

Palladium-catalyzed hydrogenation in THF of nitrophenylpyrimidine **28′** unmasked the nitro group to provide aminophenylpyrimidine **32**. Amide formation was accomplished by treatment of aniline **32** with 4-(4-methypiperazinomethyl)-benzoyl chloride (**33**) to deliver API **1**. Finally, the mesylate of **1** was readily accessed by the addition of one equivalent of methanesulfonic acid.

Meanwhile, the acid chloride side chain **33** was readily prepared from 4-(chloromethyl)benzoic acid (**34**). As shown in Scheme 4, condensation between **34** and 1-methylpiperazine provided acid **35**, which was converted to acid chloride **33** using SOCl₂.

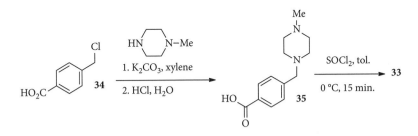

Scheme 4. Discovery Route to Prepare Side-Chain **33**

3.2 Process Synthesis

As mentioned in section 3.1, the job description of a process chemist is very different from that of a medicinal chemist. A process chemist prefers a more "convergent" approach because when the molecules reach his/her bench, extensive in vitro and in vivo assays have already been carried out. The compounds in process chemistry are quite similar to the clinical candidates.

In a patent, Novartis disclosed an alternative synthesis of **1** (Scheme 5). Instead of an S_N2 reaction of 1-methylpiperazine with benzyl chloride **34**, a reductive amination was carried out between benzaldehyde **36** and 1-methylpiperazine. Reduction of the imine was carried out by Pt/C-catalyzed hydrogenation to give acid **35**, which was readily converted to acid chloride **33**.

Subsequently, amide formation between acid chloride **33** and guanidinyl–aniline **37** to assemble amide–guanidine **38**. Pyrimidine formation was then performed by condensing **38** with known enaminone **27′** to deliver the API **1**.

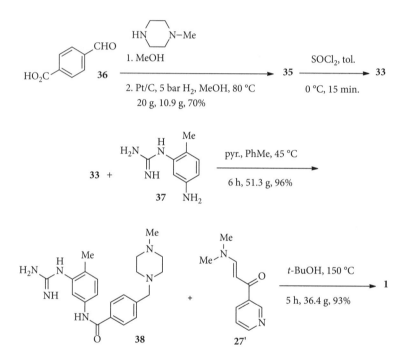

Scheme 5. Novartis' Scale-up Synthesis of Imatinib (**1**)

As soon as a major drug is approved, process chemists all over the world begin to develop alternative syntheses. Some do it because there are countries that only honor *process* patents, not *composition of matter* patents; an alternative process route will enable the inventor a different route to make and sell the drug. Others do it in anticipation of patent expiration so they can start manufacturing their generic version of the drug. Academic chemists pursue alternative synthetic routes to demonstrate the utility of the methodologies developed in their laboratories. All the efforts toward alternative syntheses of **1** were reviewed by Ley in 2013.[35]

Among the dozens of alternative synthesis, one facile synthesis is summarized here (Scheme 6).[36] Aminopyrimidine **39** was assembled by condensation of **27′** and guanidine nitrate. And enaminone **27′** was prepared from treating 1-(pyridin-3-yl) ethanone (**26′**) with DMFDMA. Meanwhile, bromobenzene **41** was prepared via bromination of 1-methyl-4-nitrobenzene (**40**). The Ullman coupling between aminopyrimidine **39** with **26′** was accomplished CuI catalysis with the aid of ligand *N,N′*-dimethylethylenediamine (DMEDA) to afford **28′**, which was reduced by hydrazine/FeCl$_3$ system to produce aniline **32**. Aniline **32** was then coupled with acid chloride **43**, prepared from acid alcohol **42**, to provide amide adduct **44**. Finally, S$_N$2 displacement of the benzyl chloride **44** with 1-methylpiperazine delivered the API **1**.

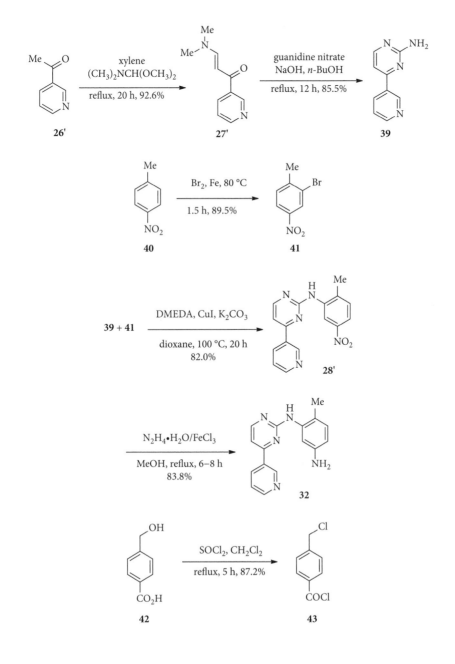

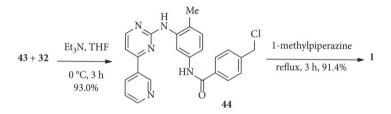

Scheme 6. Another Alternative Synthesis of Imatinib (**1**)

■ 4 CONCLUDING REMARKS

One of the challenges for targeted cancer drugs is to solve the problem of drug resistance. Tumors seem to have many pathways and they can switch course if they encounter a drug that targets their preferred pathway. Indeed, because cancer cells have many redundancies built in their growth, several pathways must be blocked to keep the tumors in check.

Because of the redundancy of cell functions, it is probably not surprising that a group of kinases, as opposed to just one single kinase, have to be blocked in order to achieve the desired effects. If only one kinase is blocked, the body most likely would find another route to achieve cell proliferation. The protein kinase inhibitors are not obliterating cancer cells despite their phenomenal benefits in shrinking tumors. Tumors seem to have more pathways than there are field mice in a meadow.

Gleevec, the golden child of targeted cancer drugs, showed drug resistance shortly after its emergence: About 15–20% of CML patients develop resistance within 3 years. The Bcr–Abl enzyme changes its shape after it wrestles with Gleevec. As a result, Gleevec keeps bumping into it but is unable to bind as it did in the original enzyme. For that 20–30% who fail Gleevec (**1**), second-line inhibitors such as dasanib (**17**) and sunitinib (**16**) are an effective salvage strategy.

As of 2014, the majority of patients diagnosed with chronic phase CML can expect to have durable responses with good quality of life. However, once the disease has progressed beyond the chronic phase, allotransplant is still the recommended treatment for all eligible patients. Unfortunately, evidence is accumulating that residual leukemia may persist even in the best responders and that therapies directed at the Bcr–Abl tyrosine kinase are not curative since they fail to eradicate the CML stem cells. Thus, the CML saga continues, and much work remains to be done.

■ 5 REFERENCES

1. Li, J. J. *Laughing Gas, Viagra, and Lipitor, The Human Stories behind the Drugs We Use*, Oxford University Press: New York, 2006, pp. 3–42.

2. Goldman, J. M. *Seminars Hemotol.* **2010**, *47*, 302–311.

3. Fischer E. H.; Krebs, E. G. *Fed. Proc.* **1966**, *25*, 1511–1520.

4. Manning, G.; Whyte, D. B.; Martinez, R.; Hunter, T.; Sudarsanam, S. *Science* **2002**, *298*, 1912–1934.

5. Vieth, M.; Sutherland, J. J.; Robertson, D. H.; Campbell, R. M. *Drug Discov. Today* **2005**, *10*, 839–846.

6. Eglen, R. M.; Reisine, T. *Exp. Opin. Drug Discov.* **2010**, *5*, 277–290.

7. Stehelin, D.; Varmus, H. E.; Bishop, J. M.; Vogt, P. K. *Nature* **1976**, *260*, 170–173.

8. Simanis, V.; Nurse, P. *Cell* **1986**, *45*, 261–268.

9. Bazell, Robert, *HER-2, The Making of Herceptin, A Revolutionary Treatment for Breast Cancer*, Random House: New York, 1998.

10. Prud'homme, Alex *The Cell Game, Samuel Waksal's Fast Money and False Promise— and the Fate of ImClone's Cancer Drug*, HarperBusiness: New York, 2004.

11. Cooke, Robert; *Dr. Folkman's War, Angiogenesis and the Struggle to Defeat Cancer*, Random House: New York, 2001.

12. Ferrara, N.; Hillan, K. J.; Gerber, H.-P.; Novotny, W. *Nature* **2004**, *3*, 391–400.

13. Goodman, L. *J. Clin. Invest.* **2004**, *113*, 934.

14. Chang, A.; Parikh, P.; Thongprasert, S. et al. *J. Thorac. Oncol.* **2006**, *1*, 847–855.

15. Pettersson, M. Sunitinib (Sutent), An angiogenesis inhibitor, in *Modern Drug Synthesis*, Li, J. J.; Johnson, D. S., Eds., Wiley: Hoboken, NJ, 2010, pp. 87–110.

16. Das, J.; Barrish, J. C. Dasatinib, a kinase inhibitor to treat chronic myelogenous leukemia, in *Analogue-Based Drug Discovery II*; Fischer, J.; Ganellin, C. R., Eds.; Wiley-VCH: Weinheim, Germany, 2010, pp. 493–509.

17. Manley, P. W.; Zimmermann, J. Setting the paradigm of targeted drugs for the treatment of cancer: Imatinib and Nilotinib, therapies for chronic myelogenous leukemia, in *Case Studies in Modern Drug Discovery and Development*; Huang, X.; Aslanian, R. G., Eds.; Wiley: Hoboken, NJ, 2012, pp. 88–102.

18. Hu, S.; Huang, Y. Sorafenib (Nexavar): a multikinase inhibitor for advanced renal cell carcinoma and unresectable hepatocellular carcinoma, in *Modern Drug Synthesis;* Li, J. J.; Johnson, D. S., Eds., Wiley: Hoboken, NJ, 2010, pp. 73–85.

19. Zhang, J.; Li, J. J. Pazopanib (Votrient): A VEGFR tyrosine kinase inhibitor for cancer, in *Modern Drug Synthesis;* Li, J. J.; Johnson, D. S., Eds., Wiley: Hoboken, NJ, 2010, pp. 111–122.

20. Cohen, P. *Nat. Rev. Drug Discov.* **2002**, *1*, 309–315.

21. Yaish, P.; Gilon, C.; Levitzki, A. *Science* **1988**, *242*, 933–935.

22. Vasella, D. *The Magic Cancer Pill, How a Tiny Orange Pill Is Rewriting Medicine History*; Harper Business: New York, 2003.

23. Nagar, B.; Bornmann, W. G.; Pellicena, P. et al. *Cancer Res.* **2002**, *62*, 4236–43.

24. Zimmermann, J.; Buchdunger, E.; Mett, H.; Meyer, T.; Lydon, N. B. *Bioorg. Med. Chem. Lett.* **1997**, *7*, 187–192.

25. Gschwind, H.-P.; Pfaar, U.; Waldmeier, F. et al. *Drug Metab. Dispos.* **2005**, *33*, 1503–1512.

26. Moen, M. D.; McKeage, K.; Plosker, G. L.; Siddiqui, M. A. A. *Drugs* **2007**, *67*, 299–320.

27. Scheinfeld, N.; Schienfeld, N. *J. Drugs Dermatol.* **2006**, *5*, 117–122.

28. Peng, B.; Dutreix, C.; Mehring, G. et al. *J. Clin. Pharmacol.* **2004**, *44*, 158–162.

29. Cohen, M. H.; Williams, G.; Johnson, J. R. et al. *Clin. Cancer Res.* **2002**, *8*, 935–942.

30. Peng, B.; Lloyd, P.; Schran, H. *Clin. Pharmacokinet.* **2005**, *44*, 879–894.

31. Cortes, J. E.; Egorin, M. J.; Guilhot, F.; Molimard, M.; Mahon, F.-X. *Leukemia* **2009**, *23*, 1537–1544.

32. Zimmermann, J. EU Pat. 0,564,409 (1993).

33. Zimmermann, J. US 5,521,184 (1996).

34. Loiseleur, O.; Kaufmann, D.; Abel, S.; Buerger, H. M.; Meisenbach, M.; Schmitz, B.; Sedelmeier, G. WTO 03066613 (2003).

35. Benjamin J. Deadman, B. J.; Hopkin, M. D.; Baxendale, I. R.; Ley, S. V. *Org. Biomol. Chem.* **2013**, *11*, 1766–1800.

36. Liu, Y.-F.; Wang, C.-L.; Bai, Y.-J.; Han, N.; Jiao, J.-P.; Qi, X.-L. *Org. Process Res. Dev.* **2008**, *12*, 490–495.

Drugs for Metabolic Diseases

6   Sitagliptin (Januvia)

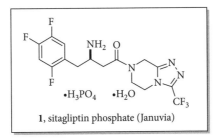

1, sitagliptin phosphate (Januvia)

USAN:	*Sitagliptin Phosphate*
Brand Name:	*Januvia (Merck)*
Molecular Weight:	*523.32 (Parent, 407.31)*
FDA Approval:	*2006*
Drug Class:	*Dipeptidyl peptidase-4 (DPP-4) inhibitor*
Indications:	*Type II Diabetes*
Mechanism of Action:	*Competitive and Reversible Dipeptidyl Peptidase IV (DPP-4) Inhibitor*

■ 1 HISTORY OF DIABETES AND DIABETIC DRUGS

Diabetes has been known since antiquity. In fact, the term "diabetes mellitus" comes from the Greek meaning "siphon and honey" due to the excess excretion (siphon or faucet) of hyperglycemic (sweetened, or honeyed) urine associated with diabetes. In ancient times, diabetes was mostly type I, which usually manifests acutely in the young, secondary to certain underlying insults (possibly infections) to the islet cells of the pancreas resulting in an absolute lack of insulin. Insulin was discovered by Banting and Best in 1921,[1,2] and insulin injection has literally saved millions of lives since then. With the wondrous efficacy that insulin bestows, type I diabetes is largely controlled because type I diabetes is insulin-dependent. However, type II diabetes, a more prevalent form of diabetes, is not insulin-dependent.

In ancient times, when nutrition was scarce and obesity was not prevalent, type II diabetes mellitus (T2DM) was extremely rare. Indeed, type II diabetes is a disease more frequently associated with maturity, obesity, and gradually increasing blood glucose concentrations, and it may be asymptomatic for some time, only discovered on routine glucose screening. In fact, with the increasing body weight of the general population of the developed world, type II diabetes is becoming an epidemic. Serious complications of diabetes include nephropathy (kidney diseases), neuropathy (nerve damage), and retinopathy (blindness). Diabetes is the most common cause of blindness and amputation in the elderly in the United States. Oral diabetes drugs are required for most type II diabetic patients.

Diabetes drugs may be classified into four categories: (a) agents that augment the supply of insulin such as sulfonylureas; (b) agents that enhance the effectiveness of insulin such as biguanides and thiazolidinediones; (c) GLP agonists; and (d) DPP4 Inhibitors. The efficacy of all the antidiabetic drugs can be monitored by measuring glycosylated hemoglobin (HaA$_{1c}$) as a long term marker of elevated blood glucose. The amount of HaA$_{1c}$ reflects the average level over the last 120 days, the life span of a red blood cell, and should remain below 7%.

1.1 Sulfonylureas

More than 20 million T2DM patients worldwide are treated with hypoglycemic sulfonylureas. Their introduction as a treatment during the 1950s represented the first reliable oral treatment of diabetes.

Janbon discovered sulfonylureas' antidiabetic effects of in 1942 by chance when he observed hypoglycemia as a side effect after giving a sulfa antibiotic to soldiers to alleviate typhoid fever.[3] That particular sulfonamide antibiotic drug

TABLE 6.1. *Important Sulfonylureas*[4]

Name	R	R¹
tolbutamide (Orinase, **3**)	–CH$_3$	–CH$_2$CH$_2$CH$_2$CH$_3$
chlorpropamide (Diabinese, **4**)	–Cl	–CH$_2$CH$_2$CH$_3$
tolazamide (Tolinase, **5**)	–CH$_3$	
acetohexamide (Dymelor, **6**)	–C(O)CH$_3$	
glibenclamide (Glynase, **7**)		
glipizide (Glucotrol, **8**)		
glimepiride (Amaryl, **9**)		

was isopropylthia-diazole (IPTD, **2**). Tolbutamide (Orinase, **3**) and chlorprop-amide (Diabinese, **4**, see Table 6.1) emerged in the 1950s. Tolbutamide (**3**), with a toluene moiety, is readily metabolized and thus required a twice-daily treatment. Chlorpropamide (**4**), on the other hand, has a chlorine substituent in place of the methyl group in tolbutamide (**3**)—therefore, chlorpropamide (**4**) is less prone to metabolization and can be taken once daily. The advantage of tolbutamide (**3**) was that it did not possess antibacterial properties, thus avoiding build-up of bacterial resistance. Unfortunately tolbutamide (**3**), marketed since 1957, was found to be associated with increased cardiac mortality and was withdrawn from the market in 1997.

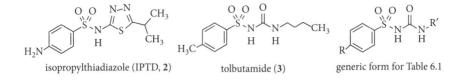

isopropylthiadiazole (IPTD, **2**)   tolbutamide (**3**)   generic form for Table 6.1

Over time, sulfonylurea use increased dramatically. Many additional sulfonyl-ureas, including tolazamide (Tolinase, **5**) and acetohexamide (Dymelor, **6**) emerged, as depicted in Table 6.2. Compounds **2–6** are the first generation sulfonylureas, whereas sulfonylureas **7–9** are the second-generation drugs.[4] They are longer-acting and highly potent. The second-generation sulfonylureas are effective at 10–100 times lower concentrations and this difference in potency is a major dis-tinction between the two generations of drugs. Today, the second-generation sul-fonylureas are the most commonly used.

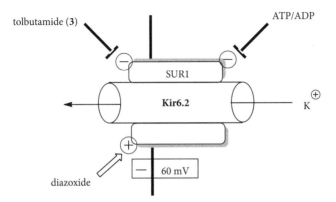

Fig. 6.1. K_{ATP} Channel in Pancreatic β-Cells (SUR = SulfonylUrea Receptor)[6]

Sulfonylureas are also known as *insulin secretagogues* because they stimulate insulin secretion by inhibiting (closing) ATP-sensitive K^+ (K_{ATP}) channels in pancreatic β-cells by binding to the sulfonylurea receptor SUR1.[4,5] Sulfonylureas promote depolarization of the β-cell membrane by closing off ATP-gated potassium channels Kir6.2 (see Fig. 6.1). However, sulfonylureas are ineffective in completely insulin-deficient patients and successful therapy likely requires at least 30% of normal β-cell function. Sulfonylureas are commonly used as an add-on to metformin (19) in treating T2DM in patients who are insufficiently controlled by metformin (19) alone; they have good efficacy and have been shown to prevent microvascular complications. However, treatment with sulfonylureas is also associated with a high frequency of hypoglycemia, increased body weight, and a high risk of secondary failure.[6]

Repaglinide (Prandin, 10), nateglinide (Starlix, 11), and mitiglinide (Glufast, 12) are non-sulfonylurea secretagogues.[7-9] They are a group of rapid-acting insulin secretion–stimulating agents also known as short-acting insulinotropic agents that can be regarded as better "sulfonylureas." For instance, nateglinide (11) is highly tissue selective with low affinity for heart and skeletal muscle. Non-sulfonylurea secretagogues 10–12 interact with the ATP-sensitive potassium channel on pancreatic β-cells. The subsequent depolarization of the β-cell opens the calcium channel, producing calcium influx and insulin secretion. The extent of insulin release is glucose dependent and diminishes at low glucose levels.

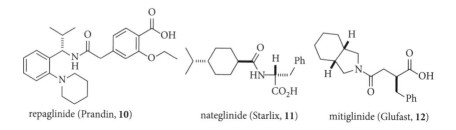

repaglinide (Prandin, 10)   nateglinide (Starlix, 11)   mitiglinide (Glufast, 12)

1.2. Biguanides

Among the pharmacological interventions to preserve the β-cells, those that lead to short-term improvement of β-cell secretion include insulin, sulfonylureas, and metformin (19). Sulfonylureas serve to increase insulin production by the pancreas. But there is limited insulin production in the pancreas of a T2DM patient. In time, the pancreas will not be able to generate insulin any longer, so there is a need for drugs to increase the insulin sensitivity of the pancreas. Biguanides and thiazolidinediones belong to this category.

A century ago, guanidine (13) was tested to determine whether it reduced blood sugar level in rabbits, but was found to be too toxic for use in humans. The same was found to be true for galegine (**14**), isolated from *Galega officinalis*, and also known as French lilac, goat's rue, or professor-weed. Synthalin A (**15**) was the first biguanide on the market in 1926, but was plagued by adverse effects. Synthalin B (**16**) was made in an effort to lower the toxicities associated with Synthalin A (**15**). However, it was also withdrawn in the 1940s due to liver and kidney toxicities.[10]

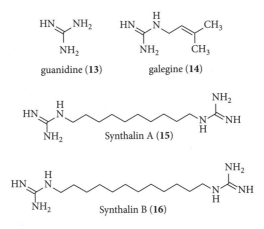

guanidine (**13**)   galegine (**14**)

Synthalin A (**15**)

Synthalin B (**16**)

Phenformin (**17**), an early biguanide, was for some time one of the few available oral agents. However, it had limited utility due to serious side effects and was withdrawn from the US and most other markets in 1977 due to high risk of lactic acidosis. Buformin (**18**), an analog of phenformin (**17**), had a somewhat better safety profile. The safest biguanide to date is metformin (Glucophage, **19**), which has 10–15 times fewer incidences of lactic acidosis and is thus safer than both phenformin (**17**) and buformin (**18**). Metformin (**19**) was first marketed in 1957 by Merck although it was first synthesized in 1922. It was reintroduced in the United States for the treatment of T2DM in 1994. Today, metformin (**19**) is one of the most commonly prescribed oral treatments for T2DM. It is preferred for obese patients unless contradicted.

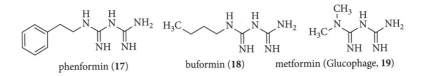

phenformin (**17**)   buformin (**18**)   metformin (Glucophage, **19**)

The MOA of metformin (**19**) has been the subject of intense investigation. Metformin has been widely thought to act as an insulin sensitizer in people with diabetes, improving the ability of insulin to stimulate glucose uptake in muscle and suppress hepatic glucose production. Like sulfonylureas, metformin (**19**) is only active in the presence of insulin. More recently, however, a new study in mice shows that inhibitory phosphorylation of acetyl-CoA carboxylases Acc1 and Acc2 by the AMP-activated protein kinase (AMPK) is essential to the ability of metformin (**19**) to improve insulin sensitivity and lower blood glucose in patients who are obese.[11]

Unlike most other antidiabetes drugs, metformin (**19**) is not bound to serum proteins and thus is not displaced by competitive binding of other drugs. The highest concentrations of metformin (**19**) are found in the gut and liver. It is not metabolized but is rapidly cleared from plasma by the kidneys. Because of its rapid clearance, metformin is usually taken 2–3 times daily. The most frequent side effect associated with metformin (**19**) is diarrhea. This kind of gastrointestinal (GI) irritation can be a sign of early lactic acidosis. Unlike sulfonylureas, hypoglycemia is *not* a complication for the use of biguanides.

1.3 PPARγ Agonists

Similar to biguanides, thiazolidinediones (TZDs) are insulin sensitizers. Thiazolidinediones are often used with other oral antidiabetic drugs, preferably with metformin or sulfonylureas.

In 1997 Sankyo and Parke-Davis began to market the first thiazolidinedione, troglitazone (Rezulin, **20**), in the United States for the treatment of T2DM. But it was voluntarily withdrawn in 2000 due to severe idiosyncratic hepatotoxicity. In 1999, the FDA approved two additional thiazolidinediones, rosiglitazone (Avandia, **21**) by GSK and pioglitazone (Actos, **22**) by Takeda and Lilly. Although they all possess the same TZD functional group as troglitazone (**20**), they are expected to be less toxic because they are more potent, thus requiring smaller doses. In 2011, the FDA severely restricted the prescription of rosiglitazone (Avandia, **21**) due to its "purported" cardiovascular side effects after a long and very controversial public debate. The FDA lifted those restrictions in 2013 after more positive data surfaced from beta analysis.

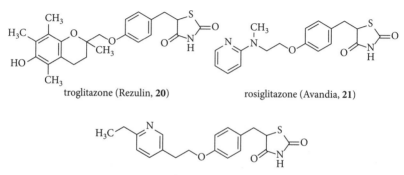

troglitazone (Rezulin, **20**)   rosiglitazone (Avandia, **21**)

pioglitazone (Actos, **22**)

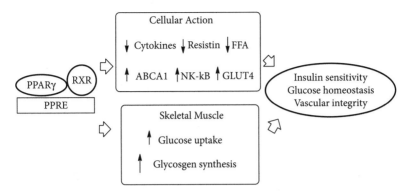

Fig. 6.2. PPAR-γ gene transcription mechanism and its biologic effects[12]

Thiazolidinediones exert their antidiabetic effects through a mechanism that involves activation (agonist) of the γ isoform of the peroxisome proliferators-activated receptor (PPAR-γ), a nuclear receptor.[12] As shown in Fig. 6.2, the process of transcription begins with the binding of ligands (endogenous or exogenous) to the PAAR-γ receptor. Ligand-bound PPAR heterodimerizes with retinoid X receptor (RXR) and this heterodimer binds to the promoter region of peroxisome proliferator response elements (PPREs) with the recruitment of co-activators. This results in the increase in transcription activities of various genes involved in diverse biological process. In addition, thiazolidinedione-induced activation of PPAR-γ alters the transcription of several genes involved in glucose and lipid metabolism and energy balance, including those that code for lipoprotein lipase, fatty acid transporter protein, adipocyte fatty acid binding protein, fatty acyl-CoA synthase, malic enzyme, glucokinase, and the GLUT4 glucose transporter.[13] Thiazolidinediones reduce insulin resistance in adipose tissue, muscle, and the liver, however, PPAR-γ is predominantly expressed in adipose tissue. It is possible that the effect of thiazolidinediones on insulin resistance in muscle and liver is promoted via endocrine signaling from adipocytes. Potential signaling factors include free fatty acids (well-known mediators of insulin resistance linked to obesity) or adipocyte-derived tumor necrosis factor-α (TNF-α), which is overexpressed in obesity and insulin resistance.

Although there are still many unknowns about the MOA of thiazolidinediones in T2DM, it is clear that these agents have the potential to benefit the full insulin resistance syndrome associated with the disease. Thiazolidinediones may also have potential benefits for the secondary complications of T2DM, such as cardiovascular diseases, despite the temporary lessening of side effects associated with rosiglitazone (Avandia, **21**).

We have summarized three classes of insulin sensitizers thus far: sulfonylureas, biguanides, and PPARγ agonists. Three additional classes of antidiabetic drugs are in use today: GLP-1 receptor agonists, SGLT-2 inhibitors, and DPP4 inhibitors. Both GLP-1 agonists and DPP4 inhibitors are incretin-based therapies.

Glucagon-like peptide-1 (GLP-1) is an incretin hormone and GLP-1 analogs or agonists are incretin mimetics. Unlike older insulin secretagogues, GLP-1 analogs have a lower risk of causing hypoglycemia. The first GLP-1 agonist exenatide was approved by the FDA in 2005. Exenatide (Byetta) is a synthetic form of exendin-4, a protein expressed in the salivary glands of the Gila monster, and shares 53% homology with human GLP-1. Since then, many GLP-1 analogs have followed:[14] Liraglutide (Victoza) was approved in 2010. Three additional GLP-1 agonists, taspoglutide, albiglutide, and lixisenatide, are now on the market as well.

Sodium-glucose–linked transporters are a family of glucose transporter found in the intestinal mucosa of the small intestine (SGLT1) and the proximal convoluted tubule (PCT) of the nephron (SGLT2). They contribute to renal glucose reabsorption. In the kidneys, 100% of the filtered glucose in the glomerulus has to be reabsorbed along the nephron (98% in PCT via SGLT2). In plasma glucose concentration that is too high (hyperglycemia), glucose is excreted in urine (glucosuria) because SGLT are saturated with the filtered monosaccharide. Inhibition of SGLT2 leads to a reduction in blood glucose levels. Therefore, SGLT2 inhibitors have potential use in the treatment of T2DM. Two SGLT2 inhibitors are now on the market for the treatment of T2DM: One is Johnson & Johnson's canagliflozin (Invokana, **23**) and the other is BMS/AstraZeneca's dapagliflozin (Farxiga, **24**).

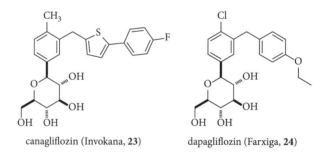

canagliflozin (Invokana, **23**)　　dapagliflozin (Farxiga, **24**)

Dipeptidyl peptidase-4 (DPP-4) inhibitors have emerged as alternatives to sulfonylureas. They show similar efficacy as sulfonylureas but with lower risk of hypoglycemia and reduction or no change in body weight, and if confirmed in humans, they may preserve islet function and thereby minimize the risk for secondary failure. Their limitation at present is the lack of long-term (>5 years) experience on durability and safety. Overall, therefore, the conclusion emerges that sulfonylureas are less desirable than DPP-4 inhibitors in management of hyperglycemia in T2DM.

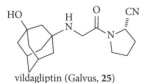 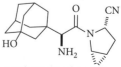

vildagliptin (Galvus, **25**)　　saxagliptin (Onglyza, **26**)

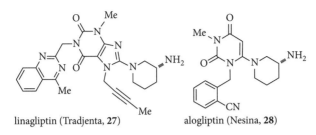

linagliptin (Tradjenta, **27**)   alogliptin (Nesina, **28**)

The approval of sitagliptin (Januvia, **1**) by the FDA in 2006 established DPP-4 inhibitors as an important new therapy for the treatment of T2DM. In addition to Januvia (**1**), four other DPP-4 inhibitors—vildagliptin (**25**), saxagliptin (**26**), lina-gliptin (**27**), and alogliptin (Nesina, **28**)—are also marketed for the treatment of T2DM. Januvia (**1**), vildagliptin (**25**), and saxagliptin (**26**) all mimic the dipeptide structure of DPP-4 substrates; while Januvia (**1**) is β-amino acid based, vildagliptin (**25**) and saxagliptin (**26**) are nitrile-based. Linagliptin (**27**), and alogliptin (Nesina, **28**) are non-peptidomimetic inhibitors.

This chapter will focus on DPP-4 inhibitors with special emphasis on Merck's Januvia (**1**), the first, and so far the best, drug in this class. Januvia (**1**) and Janumet [Januvia (**1**) plus metformin (**19**)] had combined sales of $5.7 billion in 2012.

■ 2 PHARMACOLOGY

2.1 Mechanism of Action

Both GLP-1 and glucose-dependent insulinotropic polypeptide (DIP) are "incre-tin" hormones.[15–19] They are so named because they powerfully stimulate insulin secretion and biosynthesis in response of enteric rather than the parental glucose. As shown in Fig. 6.3, GLP-1 is a peptic gut hormone with 31 amino acids. It is se-creted from the intestinal L-cells. DDP-IV is an enzyme that cleaves GLP-1 at the penultimate position from the *N*-terminus and makes it inactive.

As shown in Fig. 6.4, DPP-4 inhibitors decrease glucose by blocking the DPP-4 enzyme, which inactivates GLP-1. As a consequence, they stimulate insulin secre-tion indirectly by enhancing the action of the incretin hormones GLP-1 and glucose-dependent insulinotropic polypeptide (GIP). Since both GLP-1 and GIP stimulate insulin secretion in a glucose-dependent manner, they pose little or no risk for hypoglycemia. In addition, GLP-1 stimulates insulin biosynthesis, inhibits

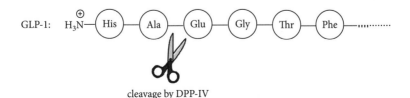

cleavage by DPP-IV

Fig. 6.3. DPP-4 Cleaves GLP-1 at the Penultimate Position from the *N*-Terminus[19]

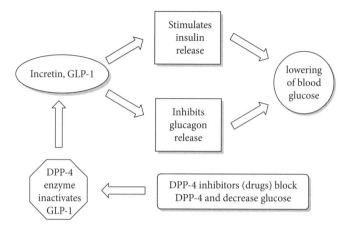

Fig. 6.4. DPP-4 inhibitors and GLP-1[nn]

TABLE 6.2. In Vitro *Potency and Selectivity of Sitagliptin (1)*[20]

Enzyme	IC_{50}	Selectivity
DPP-4	18 nM	—
QPP	>100,000 nM	>5,000
DPP8	48,000 nM	2,700
DPP9	>100,000 nM	>5,000

glucagon secretion, slows gastric emptying, reduces appetite, and stimulates the regeneration and differentiation of islet β-cells.

Thanks to the mechanism action, DPP-4 inhibitors such as Januvia (**1**) possess advantages over alternative diabetes therapies, including a lowered risk of hypoglycemia, a potential for weight loss, and a potential for the regeneration and differentiation of pancreatic β-cells.

DPP-4 is a member of a family of proteases, two of which (DPP-8 and -9) have been implicated in preclinical toxicities and suppression of T-cell activation and proliferation in some studies. In vitro, Januvia (**1**) is a potent competitive and reversible DPP-4 inhibitor that exhibits >2,600-fold in vitro selectivity over closely related enzymes such as QPP, DPP8, and DPP9 (Table 6.2).[20] Selectivity over DPP8 and DPP9 is important because a good selectivity may minimize any potential off-target side effects.

In vivo, orally administered Januvia (**1**) reduced blood glucose excursion dose dependently in an oral glucose tolerance test in lean mice. At maximally efficacious doses, a 2- to 3-fold increase of postprandial, active GLP-1 concentrations was observed. These studies demonstrate the relationship between inhibition of DPP-4, increases in active GLP-1 concentration, and an improvement in glucose tolerance after an oral glucose challenge. Inhibition of DPP-4 in rodent models for diabetes has also been shown to attenuate the decline of pancreatic β-cell function and mass. DPP-4 inhibition with Januvia (**1**) in a mouse model of T2DM resulted in improvements in glucose homeostasis and significant improvements in islet mass and β-cell function. In the same rodent model, Januvia (**1**) demonstrated improved β-cell preserving effects and superior glucose-lowering efficacy compared to glipizide (**8**), a commonly used sulfonylurea insulin secretagogue.

In phase III studies, Januvia (**1**) significantly decreases HbA_{1c} levels compared to placebo and increases the proportion of patients that achieve the American Diabetes Association (ADA) goal of <7% HbA_{1c} levels. In addition, decreases in fasting plasma glucose and 2 h postprandial glucose levels, and improvements in β-cell function have resulted from treatment with Januvia (**1**). Clinical trials comparing the Januvia (**1**) 50 mg/metformin (**19**) 1000 mg twice-daily group as opposed to the pioglitazone (**22**) group observed statistically significant ($P < 0.001$) decreases in HbA1c. There was a reduction of 1.9% in the Januvia (**1**)/metformin (**19**) group and 1.4% in the pioglitazone (**22**) group.[21]

2.2 Structure–Activity Relationship

The two lead compounds from Merck's high-throughput screening (HTS) were a proline-derived HTS lead (**29**, entry 1) and a piperazine-derived HTS lead (**30**, entry 2) as shown in Table 6.3.[20,22] Dramatically, addition of two fluorine atoms and permutation on the right-hand portion to proline **29** afforded nearly a 4,000× boost of potency for proline **31** (entry 3) in in vitro assay! A 785× increase of potency was obtained from piperazine **30** to piperazine **32** (entry 4). However, both proline **31** and piperazine **32** had negligible oral bioavailability in rats ($F_{rat} \leq 1\%$). In an attempt to remove metabolically vulnerable fragments, the right-hand portion of proline **31** was chopped off to give proline **33** (entry 5). Similarly, removal of the right-hand portion of piperazine **32** gave rise to piperazine **34** (entry 6). Unfortunately, the resulting simplified *ortho*-fluoro-homophenylalanine amides **33** and **34** also possess low oral bioavailabilities in rats due to metabolic instability of the thiazolidine and piperazine rings, respectively.

At this stage, both the proline series and the piperazine series began to coalesce to fused triazole **35** (entry 7) after extensive SAR using a variety of fused heterocycles in an effort to improve metabolic stability and DPP-4 potency. While triazole **35** had similar potency to that of thiazoline **33** and piperazine **34**, it had marked improvement of metabolic stability in rat hepatocytes although its oral bioavailability in rats was still low. In fact, while ethyl analog **35** suffered from poor oral bioavailability in both the rat model and the rhesus monkey model, it showed fair oral bioavailability in the dog model. Presumably, triazole **35**'s low oral bioavailability in rats was a result of CYP450 oxidation of the diflurobenzene ring on the left and the ethyl group. Installing the third fluorine on the benzene ring and replacing the ethyl group with a trifluoromethyl group delivered Januvia (**1**) (entry 8) with an oral bioavailability of 76% in rats as well as good potency against DPP-4.

TABLE 6.3. *The SAR leading to sitagliptin (1)*[20]

Entry	Structure	IC$_{50}$ (nM)
1		1,900
2		11,000
3		0.48
4		14
5		270
6		139
7		231
8		18

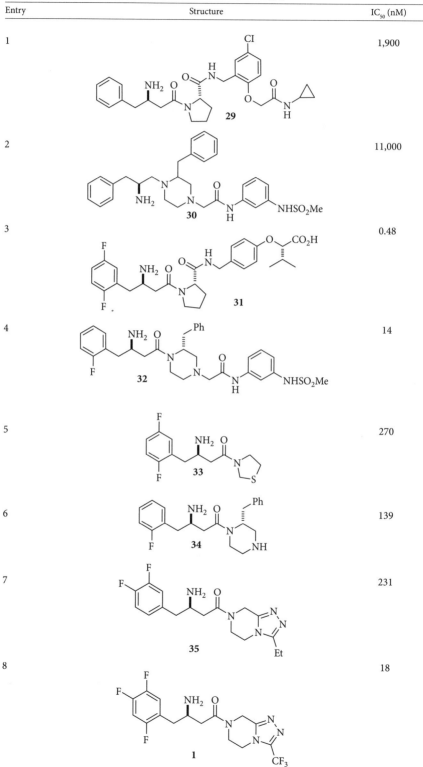

Overall, Januvia (**1**) was superior to other fused heterocycle derivatives in terms of potency, off-target selectivity, and preclinical pharmacokinetic (PK) profile.

2.3 Bioavailability, Metabolism, and Toxicology

In humans, Januvia (**1**) is rapidly absorbed with significant inhibition of plasma DPP-4 activity being seen within 5 min of administration.[23] Its oral biovailability in humans is generally high (~87%), as shown in Table 6.4. Januvia (**1**) has a maximum (peak) plasma concentration (C_{max}) of approximately 1000 nmol/L. Its total exposure, represented AUC, is approximately 10 nmol•h/L.

Consistent with its mechanism in blocking peptide receptors found primarily on endothelial membranes, the volume of distribution of Januvia (**1**) is modest, 2.01 L/kg, that is, 151 L for an average patient (75 kg). At steady state, the exposure of Januvia (**1**) increases by ~14% compared to exposures after a single dose. Januvia (**1**) exhibits relatively low reversible plasma protein binding and is widely distributed into tissue.

Similar to linagliptin (**27**), and alogliptin (**28**), Januvia (**1**) does not undergo appreciable metabolism in vivo in humans; around 80% of the dose is eliminated unchanged as the parent compound. For Januvia (**1**), the limited metabolism produces six metabolites in trace amounts (each accounting for <1% to 7% of Januvia-related material in plasma), with in vitro studies indicating that the primary enzyme responsible is CYP3A4 with a lesser contribution from CYP2C8.[24] Three of these metabolites—M1 (**36**), M2 (**37**), and M5 (**38**)—are active, but are not expected to contribute to the pharmacodynamic profile of Januvia (**1**) because of the combination of low plasma concentration and low affinity for DPP-4. None of the inhibitors have been reported to have any significant inhibitory activity on a panel of different enzymes, including the CYP450 enzymes.

TABLE 6.4. *Human Pharmacokinetic Properties of sitagliptin (1)*[23]

Bioavailability (F)	87%
C_{max}	817±250 nmol/L
Area Under the Curve	
(AUC$_{0-\infty}$)	10 nmol•h/L
Volume of Distribution (V_d)	2.01 L/Kg
Protein Binding	38%
T_{max}	1–4 h
$t_{1/2}$	12 h

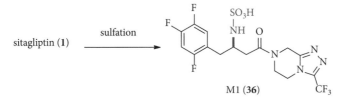

M1 (**36**)

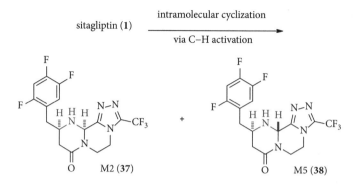

The major elimination pathway for Januvia (**1**) in humans is excretion of parent compound in urine. Consequently, increased exposure (2- to 4-fold) is observed in patients with impaired renal function. In vitro data indicate that Januvia (**1**) is unlikely to be involved in any DDIs with the CYP450 enzyme system. DDI studies with Januvia (**1**) demonstrated no meaningful alterations of the pharmacokinetic profiles of other co-administered diabetes medications, including metformin (**19**), rosiglitazone (**21**), and glyburide. Indeed, no meaningful DDI has been found in patients treated with 83 different co-administered drugs in clinical trials.

Januvia (**1**) 100 mg/day is well tolerated in patients with T2DM, with an overall profile similar to placebo. In dose-escalation studies, a single 100 mg oral dose of Januvia (**1**) was shown to inhibit DPP-4 by >80% over 24 h in healthy adults and Januvia (**1**) was well tolerated up to a single dose of 800 mg/day and multiple doses of 400 mg/day for 28 days. In all, the safety of Januvia (**1**) is on par with that of placebo. There was a low incidence of hypoglycemia in Januvia (**1**) treated patients, which is consistent with its glucose-dependent MOA.

In 24-week add-on studies with metformin (**19**), pioglitazone (**20**), glimepiride (**9**), or glimepiride (**9**)/metformin (**19**), the addition of Januvia (**1**) 100 mg/day resulted in greater reductions in HbA$_{1c}$ and a greater proportion of patients reaching a target HbA$_{1c}$ of <7% compared to the respective monotherapies.

■ 3 SYNTHESES

3.1 Discovery Synthesis

Logistically, the medicinal chemistry synthesis was accomplished by amide formation between carboxylic acid **39** and piperazine **40**.[20,22]

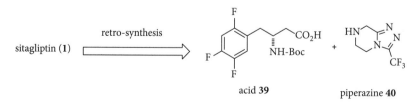

acid **39**   piperazine **40**

Merck chemists first applied Schöllkopf's bis-lactim methodology[25] and prepared α-amino acid **43** was realized by two-step application. Schöllkopf's bis-lactim **41**, which may be viewed as a masked valine, was deprotonated with *n*-BuLi and quenched by benzylbromide **42**. Protection of amine with (Boc)$_2$O was followed by hydrolysis and treatment with diazomethane to produce diazo-compound **44**. Treatment of diazo-compound **44** with silver benzoate and hydrolysis provided carboxylic acid **39**. Amide formation between carboxylic acid **39** and piperazine **40**, promoted by 1-ethyl-3-(3-dimethylaminopropyl)carbodiimide (EDC, aka, EDAC, or EDCI), was followed by removal of Boc delivered Januvia (**1**).

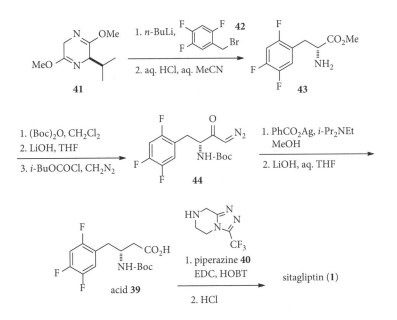

As far as triazole-piperazine **40** was concerned, Merck's process chemists involved early during the project to improve the literature procedure published by Pott.[26] After two iterations,[27,28] a robust practical manufacturing route suitable for large-scale preparation was developed.[28] Selective sequential condensation of 35% aqueous hydrazine with 1 equiv ethyl trifluoroacetate and 1 equiv chloroacetyl chloride prepared bis-amide **45**. In one pot, cyclodehydration of bis-amide **45** using phosphorus oxychloride produced the key intermediate chloromethyloxadiazole. Treating **46** with ethylenediamine in methanol gave amidine **48** via intermediate **47**. Mechanistically, this transformation is reminiscent of the Sternbach reaction to synthesize benzodiazepines. Rather than S$_N$2 displacement of the "benzyl" chloride, the crucial nucleophilic methanol proceeds as a nucleophile, adds to the oxadiazole ring, and expels the chloride to afford oxadiazoline **47**. The nucleophilic addition of ethylenediamine to the *oxo*-olefin triggered a cascade reaction that ends with amidine **48**. Eventually, cyclodehydration of amidine **48** then delivered triazole-piperazine **40**. The overall yield of this manufacturing process is 52%, nearly double that of the original route. Importantly, use of 1 equiv aqueous hydrazine, which is completely consumed in the first step, results in safer operating conditions and cleaner waste streams.

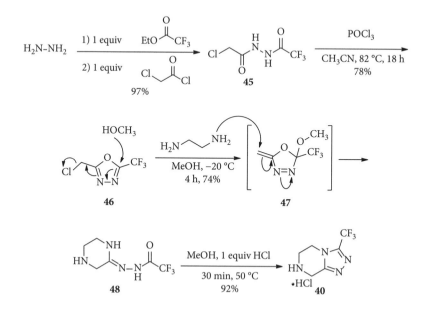

3.2 Process/Manufacturing Synthesis

Many aspects of the first-generation synthesis made it suitable for the large-scale preparation of Januvia (**1**). Nevertheless, the first-generation route relies on an inefficient method of creating the β-amino acid moiety via asymmetric hydrogenation of a β-keto ester intermediate. To overcome this drawback and achieve a more efficient and environmentally friendly synthesis, the Merck Process Research team focused their efforts on asymmetric hydrogenation of N-protected/unprotected enamine substrates to directly set up the desired stereochemistry as well as the functionality of Januvia (**1**).

To achieve this ultimate goal, a short, concise synthesis of dehydrositagliptin **53** was developed. The approach used to prepare **53** capitalized on the ability of Meldrum's acid to act as an acyl anion equivalent. This process involves activation of **49** by formation of a mixed anhydride with pivaloyl chloride, in the presences of Meldrum's acid, i-Pr₂NEt, and a catalytic amount of dimethylaminopyridine (DMAP) to form **50**. The formation of β-keto amide **52** occurred via degradation of **50** to an oxo-ketene intermediate **51** which was trapped with piperazine **40**. Without workup, NH₄OAc and methanol were mixed with the crude reaction mixture to furnish dehydrositagliptin **53**, which contains, save two hydrogen atoms,

the entire structure of Januvia (**1**). Importantly, **53** was prepared in an easily oper-
ated one-pot process in 82% overall isolated yield with 99.6 wt% purity through
a simple filtration, thereby eliminating the need for aqueous workup and minimizing waste generation.

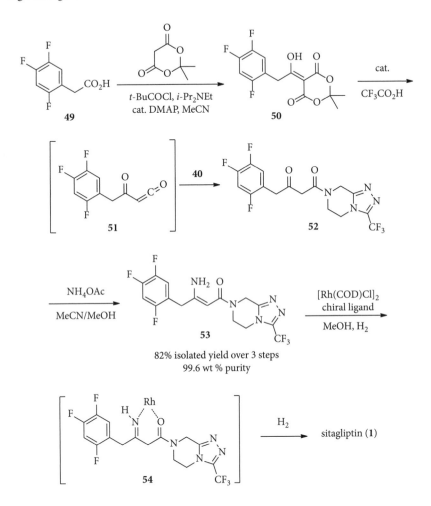

To explore the feasibility of the unprecedented asymmetric hydrogenation of
unprotected enamines, a focused pilot screen on substrate **53** with a relatively small
set of commercially available chiral bisphosphines in combination with Ir, Ru, and
Rh salts was performed.[29] Metal catalysts Ir, Ru, and Rh were selected for this
screen due to their demonstrated performance in asymmetric hydrogenations. It
was astonishing that the screening results not only showed a trend of enantioselec-
tivities, but also resulted in a very direct hit. While Ir and Ru catalysts gave poor
results, [Rh(COD)$_2$OTf], in particular with ferrocenyl-based JOSIPHOS-type catalysts, afforded both high conversion and enantioselectivity. Further screening

revealed that other ligands not limited to the ferrocenyl structural class could effect this transformation with high enantioselectivity.[30] Using [Rh(COD)Cl]$_2$ as the catalyst, several ligands provided the highest levels of enantioselectivity for reduction of **54**. In summary, an overall consideration of yield, enantioselectivity, reaction rate, and ligand cost, led to a decision to pursue the [Rh(COD)Cl]$_2$-t-Bu-JOSIPHOS combination for further development to deliver a viable hydrogenation process for the commercial manufacture of **1**.

This highly efficient, asymmetric synthesis[31] of Januvia (**1**) has been implemented on manufacturing scale. The entire synthesis is carried out with a minimum number of operations: a one-pot process affords crystalline dehydrositagliptin (**53**) in >99.6 wt%; the highly enantioselective hydrogenation of **53** in the presence of as low as 0.15 mol% t-Bu JOSIPHOS-Rh(I) gives **1** in high yield and >95% ee. After the precious metal catalyst is selectively recovered/removed from the process stream, **1** is isolated as a free base, which is further converted to the final pharmaceutical form, a monohydrate phosphate salt, in >99.9% purity and >99.9% ee. The use of low Rh(I) loading for the asymmetric hydrogenation in combination with an ease of recovery of the precious rhodium metal made this process highly cost-effective. The overall yield of this process is up to 65%.

Many alternative process routes have been patented. In one example, β-keto-ester **55** was used as the key intermediate.[32] Ketone **55** was converted to it corresponding enamine, which was then protected as enamide **56**. An asymmetric hydrogenation was accomplished using TangPhos as the catalyst to form an Rh-complex **57** to produce amide **58** in excellent selectivity. Switching acetic amide to a Boc-protected amine provided amino acid **59**, which can be readily converted to Januvia (**1**).

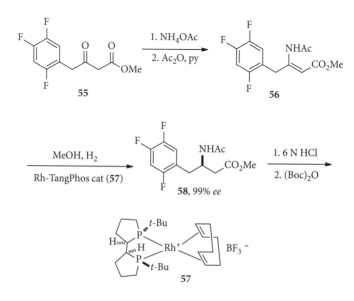

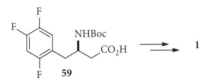

■ 4 CONCLUDING REMARKS

Diabetes has become a global epidemic, affecting more and more people. In addition, all the medicines discussed can only alleviate the symptoms; none of them is a *cure*.

At Sir Fredrick Banting Square in London, Ontario, an eternal flame—the flame of hope—is burning. When a cure for diabetes is found, it will be extinguished by the researcher(s) who discovered the cure.

■ 5 REFERENCES

1. Bliss, M. *The Discovery of Insulin*, 2nd ed., University of Toronto Press: Toronto, 1982.

2. Campbell, W. R. *Can. Med. Assoc. J.* **1962**, *17*, 1055–1061.

3. Janbon, M. *Montpellier Méd.* **1942**, *441*, 21–22.

4. Seino, S.; Zhang, C.-L.; Shibasaki, T. *J. Diabetes Invest.* **2010**, *1*, 37–39.

5. Seino, S.; Takahashi H.; Takahashi, T.; Shibasaki, T. *Diab. Obes. Metab.* **2012**, *14(Suppl. 1)*, 9–13.

6. Ahrén, B. *Curr. Diabetes Rep.* **2011**, *11*, 83–90.

7. Phillippe, H. M.; Wargo, K. A. *Exp. Opin. Pharmacother.* **2013**, *14*, 2133–2144.

8. Malaisse, W. J. *Treatments Endocrinol.* **2003**, *2*, 401–414.

9. Dornhorst, A. *Lancet* **2001**, *358*, 1709–1716.

10. Sneader, W. *Drug Discovery, A History*, Wiley: Chichester, UK, 2005, p. 276.

11. Fullerton, M. D.; Galic, S.; Marcinko, K. et al. *Nature Med.* **2013**, *19*, 1649–1654.

12. Kota, B. P.; Huang, T. H.; Roufogalis, B. D. *Pharmacol. Res.* **2005**, *51*, 85–94.

13. Gupta, D.; Kono, T.; Evans-Molina, C. *Diabetes Obes. Metab.* **2010**, *12*, 1036–1047.

14. Garber, A. J. *Exp. Opin. Invest. Drugs* **2012**, *21*, 45–57.

15. Peters, J.-U.; Mattei, P. Dipeptidyl peptidase IV inhibitors for the treatment of type II diabetes, In *Analogue-Based Drug Discovery II*, Fischer, J.; Ganellin, C. R., Eds., Wiley-VCH: Weinheim, Germany, 2010, pp. 109–134.

16. Deacon, C. F.; Holst, J. J. *Exp. Opin. Pharmacother.* **2013**, *14*, 2047–2058.

17. Gallwitz, B. *Diab. Metab. Synd. Obes. Targets Ther.* **2013**, *6*, 1–9.

18. Edmondson, S. D.; Xu, F.; Armstrong, J. D., III Sitagliptin (Januvia): a treatment for type II diabetes, in *Modern Drug Synthesis*, Li, J. J.; Johnson, D. S., Eds., Wiley: Hoboken, NJ, 2010, pp. 125–44.

19. Parmee, E. R.; SinhaRoy, R.; Xu, F.; Givand, J. C.; Rosen, L. A. Discovery and development of the DPP-4 inhibitor Januvia (sitagliptin), in *Case Studies in Modern Drug Discovery and Development*, Huang, X.; Aslanian, R. G., Eds., Wiley: Hoboken, NJ, 2012, pp. 10–140.

20. Kim, D.; Wang, L.; Beconi, M. et al. *J. Med. Chem.* **2005**, *48*, 141–151.

21. Wainstein, J.; Katz, L.; Engel, S. S.; et al. *Diabetes Obes. Metab.* **2012**, *14*, 409–418.

22. Xu, J.; Ok, H. O.; Gonzalez, E. J. et al. *Bioorg. Med. Chem. Lett.* **2004**, *14*, 4759–4762.

23. Golightly, L. K.; Drayna, C. C.; McDermott, M. T. *Clin. Pharmacokinet* **2012**, *51*, 501–514.

24. Vincent, S. H.; Reed, J. R.; Bergman, A. J. et al. *Drug Metab. Dispos.* **2007**, *35*, 533–538.

25. Schöllkopf, U.; Groth, U.; Deng, C. *Angew. Chem. Int. Ed.* **1981**, *20*, 798–799.

26. Nelson, P. J.; Potts, K. T. *J. Org. Chem.* **1962**, *27*, 3243–3248.

27. Hansen, K. B.; Balsells, J.; Dreher, S. et al. *Org. Process Res. Dev.* **2005**, *9*, 634–639.

28. Balsells, J.; DiMichele, L.; Liu, J.; Kubryk, M.; Hansen, K.; Armstrong, J. D. III *Org. Lett.* **2005**, *7*, 1039–1042.

29. Ikemoto, N.; Tellers, D. M.; Dreher, S. D. et al. *J. Am. Chem. Soc.* **2004**, *126*, 3048–3049.

30. For detailed mechanistic studies, see Xu, F.; Armstrong, J. D. III; Zhou, G. X. et al. *J. Am. Chem. Soc.* **2004**, *126*, 13002–13009.

31. For preliminary communication, see Hsiao, Y.; Rivera, N. R.; Rosner, T. et al. *J. Am. Chem. Soc.* **2004**, *126*, 9918–9919.

32. Wu, S.; Yu, B.; Delice, A.; Zhu, J. US 8, 278, 486 (2012).

CNS Drugs

7

Duloxetine Hydrochloride (Cymbalta)

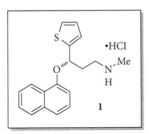

1

USAN:	*Duloxetine Hydrochloride*
Brand Name:	*Cymbalta (Eli Lilly)*
Molecular Weight:	*277.41 (Parent, 333.88)*
FDA Approval:	*1994*
Drug Class:	*Selective Serotonin and Norepinephrine Reuptake Inhibitor (SNRI) Antidepressant*
Indications:	*Major Depressive Disorder, Generalized Anxiety Disorder, Diabetic Peripheral Neuropathic Pain, Fibromyalgia, and Chronic Musculoskeletal Pain*
Mechanism of Action:	*Serotonin and Norepinephrine Reuptake Inhibitor (SNRI)*

■ 1 HISTORY OF DEPRESSION AND ANTIDEPRESSANTS

"To live is to suffer, to survive is to find some meaning in the suffering." Nietzsche's words ring true to many. Depression is romanticized at times due to its association with poets and artists, but in reality depression, especially major depressive disorder (MDD), can be debilitating.

There are two types of depression: MDD and bipolar, also known as manic–depressive illness. Severe changes in mood is the primary clinical manifestation of both disorders. MDD presents as feelings of intense sadness and despair with little drive for either socialization or communication; physical changes such as insomnia, anorexia, and sexual dysfunction can also occur. Mania is manifested by excessive elation, irritability, insomnia, hyperactivity, and impaired judgment. It may afflict as much as 1% of the population.

MDD is among the most common psychiatric disorders in humans, affecting up to 10% of men and 20% of women over the course of their lives. Among those affected, 28% experience a moderate degree of functional impairment, while 59% experience severe reductions in their normal functional ability. About 19 million

Americans suffer from depression per year. In terms of disease burden, MDD ranks as the fourth most costly illness in the world, with estimated annual costs of depression in the US amounting to approximately $43.7 billion.

While we all agree that depression exists, we do not all agree on the causes of depression. The exact causes of depression are not definitively known. However, in the 1950s, it was observed that in addition to its other pharmacological properties, reserpine (a *Rauwolfia* alkaloid) induced a depressive state in normal patients and also depleted levels of neurotransmitters such as norepinephrine (NE) and serotonin (5-HT). This observation and others led to the hypothesis that the biological basis of major mood disorders may include abnormal monoamine neurotransmission. Substances such as NE, serotonin, and dopamine (DA) mediate neurotransmission. These substances are released from presynaptic neurons, cross the synaptic gap, and interact with receptors on the postsynaptic cells. The synthesis, transmission, and processing of these neurotransmitters provide a number of points of intervention through which a pharmacological agent may affect transmission. The monoamine hypothesis of depression has held true thus far and manipulation of neurotransmission has been the mainstay of antidepressant therapy for more than half a century. Recently, the serotonin/NE link hypothesis has gained momentum as well, as manifested by the popularity of Cymbalta (**1**).

Several interventions for MDD are possible, including (1) inhibiting enzymes that synthesize neurotransmitters, (2) preventing neurotransmitter storage in synaptic vesicles, (3) blocking the release of the neurotransmitter into the synaptic gap, (4) inhibiting neurotransmitter degradation, (5) blocking neurotransmitter reuptake (removal), (6) agonism or antagonism of the postsynaptic receptor, and (7) inhibiting signal transduction within the postsynaptic cell. Pharmacological agents have been identified which affect all of these processes; however, the mainstays of antidepressant therapy have been agents that affect neurotransmitter degradation and reuptake.

1.1 Monoamine Oxidase Inhibitors

Discovered in 1951 by Hoffmann-La Roche, antibacterial isoniazid (**2**) was credited with dramatically reducing the incidence of tuberculosis in the United States. In 1952, iproniazid (Marsilid, **3**) was initially prepared, also by Hoffmann-La Roche, as an anti-tuberculosis drug to improve upon isoniazid (**2**)'s profile. Kline at Rockland State Hospital observed that iproniazid (**3**) showed a mood-enhancing effect on TB patients.[1-4] From then on, iproniazid (**3**) was widely prescribed "off-label" (i.e., for a use not approved by the FDA) as an antidepressant. However, hepatoxicity (possibly because the presence of the oxidizable group hydrazine) was observed with iproniazid (**3**) and it was withdrawn from the US market in 1961.

Mood elevation was assumed to result from the accumulation of amines such as NE and serotonin in the central nervous system (CNS). It was later found that both were monoamine oxidase inhibitors (MAOIs). Monoamine deoxidase (MAO) is a flavin-containing enzyme found in the mitochondria of neurons and other cell types. It oxidatively deaminates naturally occurring sympathomimetic monoamines such as NE, dopamine, and serotonin within the pre-synapse. MAOIs and their use in the treatment of depressed patients was a major milestone in modern psychiatry. Due to their unfavorable efficacy-safety profile, they have been replaced—initially by tricyclic antidepressants (their use has been in decline as well) and now largely by selective serotonin reuptake inhibitors (SSRIs).

At present, three MAOIs are still in use: phenelzine (Nardil, **4**), tranylcypromine (Parnate, **5**), and isocarboxazid (Marplan, **6**). All three MAOIs are non-selective MAOIs, inactivating both Type A and Type MAOs. They inhibit MOA irreversibly so they are also known as suicide inhibitors. They are classified as first-generation MAOIs.

One of the side effects of MAOIs is hypertension, also secondary to catecholamine excess, usually in association with the consumption of other catechols or catechol precursors such as tyramine (the so-called cheese effect). In an effort to develop safer MAOIs—at least away from the hypertensive liability, two subtypes of the MAO receptor have been identified, MAO-A and MAO-B. An irreversible selective MAO-B inhibitor, selegiline (Eldepryl, **7**), has been used to treat movement disorders caused by Parkinson's disease. Selegiline (**7**) is known as the second-generation MAOI. (Interestingly, selegiline (**7**) is metabolized to L-methamphetamine and L-amphetamine in humans.[5,6])

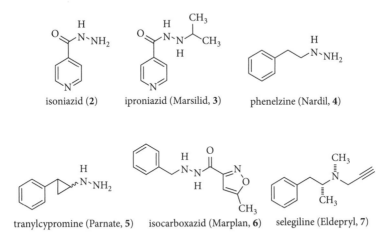

isoniazid (**2**)   iproniazid (Marsilid, **3**)   phenelzine (Nardil, **4**)

tranylcypromine (Parnate, **5**)   isocarboxazid (Marplan, **6**)   selegiline (Eldepryl, **7**)

In addition to older, irreversible nonselective (first-generation) MAOIs **4–6** and the second generation irreversible selective drug selegiline (**7**), there are third-generation MAOIs that are newer, reversible selective MAOIs. These include moclobemide (Manerix, **8**), toloxatone (Humoryl, **9**), and brofaromine (Consonar, **10**), which are also known as reversible inhibitors of MOA-A (RIMAs).

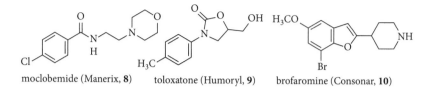

moclobemide (Manerix, 8)   toloxatone (Humoryl, 9)   brofaromine (Consonar, 10)

Both moclobemide (8) and brofaromine (10) are effective treatments for depression; they seem to be as effective as phenelzine (4) and tranylcypromine (5). Selegiline (7) has significant antidepressive efficacy, but only at high doses where there is likely to be a loss of selective inhibition of MAO-B.[7] Moclobemide (8) has a more favorable overall tolerability profile than tranylcypromine (5), with a lower incidence of adverse effects. In particular, the lack of behavioral toxicity, minimal potentiation for the tyramine pressor response, and safety in overdose are clear-cut advantages of RIMAs over older MAOIs.

Currently, the MAOIs only play a subordinate role as second-line treatments. They have been largely replaced by tricyclic antidepressants (TCAs), SSRIs, and serotonin and norepinephrine reuptake inhibitors (SNRIs).

1.2 Tricyclic Antidepressants

Imipramine (Tofranil, 12) was prepared by Geigy as an analog of an antipsychotic chlorpromazine (Thorazine, 11).[8] In 1958, imipramine's (Tofranil, 12) pronounced mood elevation in tuberculosis patients was disclosed, thus heralding the arrival of TCAs.

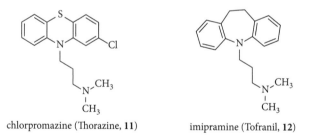

chlorpromazine (Thorazine, 11)   imipramine (Tofranil, 12)

Imipramine (12) works by inhibiting NE reuptake at the adrenergic endings, and serotonin to a lesser extent. In general, the MOA of TCAs is inhibition of re-uptake of the biogenic amines. When a neurotransmitter is released from a cell, it has only a short period of time to relay its signal before it is either metabolized by MAO or reabsorbed into the cell. All of the TCAs potentiate the actions of NE, serotonin, and to a lesser extent, dopamine. However, the potency and selectivity for inhibiting the uptake of these amines vary greatly among the agents.

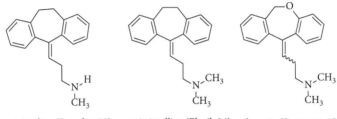

nortriptyline (Pamelor, **13**)   amitriptylline (Elavil, **14**)   doxepin (Sinequan, **15**)

In addition to imipramine (Tofranil, **12**), TCAs **13–15** are known as the first-generation TCAs to work by a similar mechanism. The so-called second-generation TCAs (also known as atypical antidepressants) include amoxapine (Asendin, **16**) and clomipramine (Anafranil, **17**).

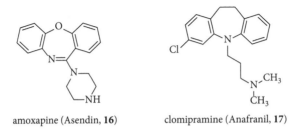

amoxapine (Asendin, **16**)   clomipramine (Anafranil, **17**)

Structurally different from the TCAs, amoxapine (Asendin, **16**) is primarily a norepinephrine reuptake inhibitor, clinically as effective as imipramine (**12**) although it may be slightly more effective in relieving accompanying anxiety and agitation. Unfortunately, like most TCAs, overdose of amoxapine (**16**) can result in fatality.

Structurally a TCA, clomipramine (**17**) exerts inhibitory effects on serotonin (5-HT) reuptake. Its metabolite demethyl-clomipramine also inhibits NE reuptake. Therefore, is classified as an SNRI, the same class as Cymbalta (**1**). In addition to being prescribed as a TCA, clomipramine (**17**) has been prescribed to treat obsessive-compulsive disorder (OCD) for many years with about 45–75% of patients responding favorably. Because clomipramine (**17**) has an additional chlorine atom in comparison to imipramine (**12**), its half-life is twice as long. The value of $t_{1/2}$ for clomipramine (**17**) is 20–40 h whereas $t_{1/2}$ for imipramine (**12**) is 10–25 h, a testimony to the metabolism-resistant property of a chlorine atom in place of a proton.

Because all TCAs are lipophilic, they are well absorbed after oral administration. They distribute widely in tissues of the body. The most prominent metabolism is demethylation of the ubiquitous dimethylamine to give the corresponding secondary amines that are also active. TCAs have long half-lives, frequently more than 24 h, which allows once-daily dosing. This feature is a major factor in achieving compliance and thus therapeutic success.

Even though these TCA agents are efficacious in their management of depression, they have significant side effects and toxicities (e.g., flushing, sweating, orthostatic hypotension, constipation). Some side effects are due to their α-adrenergic blocking activity. All the TCAs are especially toxic in overdose, producing cardiac effects and seizures.

1.3 Selective Serotonin Reuptake Inhibitors

The search for less toxic monoamine reuptake inhibitors led to the development of the safer antidepressants known as SSRIs.[9-13] Initially, AB Astra discovered and marketed zimelidine (Zelmid, **18**), the prototype of the SSRIs. Unfortunately, a rare but serious side effect, Guillain-Barré syndrome, surfaced after zimeldine (**18**) was approved in 1982 and administered in a large patient base. AB Astra pulled it off the market one year later.

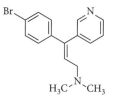

zimelidine (Zelmid, **18**)

Using diphenhydramine (Benadryl, **19**) as the starting point, Elli Lilly discovered fluoxetine hydrochloride (Prozac, **20**).[14] It was approved by the FDA in 1988 and rapidly revolutionized the treatment of depression thanks largely to its superior safety profile. Prozac transformed debilitating depression into a manageable disease for many patients. In fact, unlike the previous relatively toxic TCAs, which were prescribed primarily by psychiatrists, the much safer Prozac was frequently prescribed by non-psychiatrists and general practitioners, taking the field of psychiatry more into the open. In 2000, Prozac was the most widely prescribed antidepressant drug in the United States with worldwide sales of $2.58 billion.

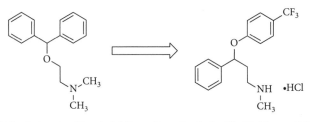

diphenhydramine (Benadryl, **19**)   fluoxetine hydrochloride (Prozac, **20**)

After Prozac's (**20**) tremendous success, many additional SSRIs soon followed. Pfizer's sertraline hydrochloride (Zoloft, **21**) and GSK's paroxetine hydrochloride

(Paxil, **22**) were launched in the Unites States in 1992. Compared to Prozac (**20**), Zoloft (**21**) has a shorter duration of action and fewer CNS-activating side effects such as nervousness and anxiety. Paxil (**22**)'s relatively benign side-effect profile favors its use in elderly patients.

Lundbeck's racemic citalopram (Celexa, **23**) was approved by the FDA in 1998 and its single (S)-enantiomer, escitalopram (Lexapro, **24**), became available in the United States in 2002. Solvy's (now part of Abbvie) fluvoxamine (Luvox, **25**) was approved by the FDA in 1994. Merck KGaA/Forest's vilazodone (Viibryn, **26**), approved by the FDA in 2011, is a combined SSRI (5-HT) and partial agonist at serotonin 1A (5-HT$_{1A}$) receptors.[15] Vilazodone (**26**) exhibits a ~300-fold selectivity for the serotonin over the NE reuptake and is inactive (or shows negligible activity) against the other 5-HT receptors, including 5-HT$_{1D}$, 5-HT$_{2A}$, and 5-HT$_{2C}$.

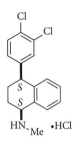

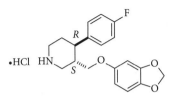

sertraline hydrochloride (Zoloft, **21**)   paroxetine hydrochloride (Paxil, **22**)

citalopram (Celexa, **23**)   escitalopram (Lexapro, **24**)

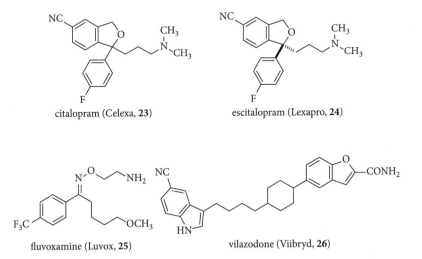

fluvoxamine (Luvox, **25**)   vilazodone (Viibryd, **26**)

Pharmacologically, SSRIs block neuronal transport of serotonin leading to increased synaptic serotonin, which in turn stimulates a large number of postsynaptic serotonin receptor types including 5-HT1B, 5-HT1D, 5-HT3 and 5-HT2C (there are 14 subtypes of serotonin receptors). Stimulation of different receptors leads to analgesia, gastrointestinal side effects and sexual dysfunction (5-HT3), and agitation and restlessness (5-HT2C). There is also a negative-feedback mechanism (by action of 5-HT1A and 1D) that suppresses serotonin neurons and decreases neuronal release of serotonin.[16]

SSRIs **20–26** differ from the older TCAs in that they selectively inhibit the reuptake of serotonin into the presynaptic nerve terminals and therefore enhance synaptic concentrations of serotonin and facilitate serotonergic transmission. This increased neurotransmission and the elevated synaptic levels of serotonin alleviate the symptoms and possibly the etiology of depression. Relative to the TCAs they have a favorable side-effect profile and are much safer in overdose. However, they are generally not more efficacious than the TCAs, they exhibit a marked delay in onset of action (it generally takes 2–3 weeks for the efficacy to manifest), and they have their own set of side effects resulting from the nonselective stimulation of serotonergic receptor sites.

SSRIs are now the first-line treatment for depression but their efficacy in major depression is no greater than TCAs. Some studies have shown that TCAs such as clomipramine (**17**) may have greater efficacy than that SSRIs such as paroxetine (**22**) and citalopram (**23**). Although they are not more efficacious than some TCAs, SSRIs possess much better safety profiles with fewer adverse effects and thus show higher compliance rates.

1.4 Serotonin and Norepinephrine Reuptake Inhibitors

Due to genetic disparities, each individual responds differently to different types of antidepressants. Many second- and third-generation antidepressants have been discovered, providing a wide variety of choice in managing depression.

The monoamine hypothesis advanced in 1965 postulated that depression is a consequence of decrease of amines such as serotonin (5-HT) and NE. Indeed TCAs inhibit the reuptake of both 5-HT and NE. Relatively selective NE reuptake inhibitors have clear antidepressant efficacy. Increasing NE neurotransmission via blockade of α2-adrenoceptors improves depressive symptoms. Finally, electroconvulsive therapy (ECT) has been shown to increase the release of NE. All this evidence indicates that stopping the removal of NE will have a beneficial effect on the mood. This is why SNRIs are also known as "boosted" SSRIs by some or "better tolerated tricyclic antidepressants" by others. SNRIs have a spectrum of ratios of 5-HT and NE, which are responsible for their diverse pharmacological effects.[17]

In 1993, venlafaxine (Effexor, **27**) was the first SNRI to be introduced. Effexor was Wyeth's largest selling drug with over $3 billion in sales in 2004. Today, Effexor (**27**) has become a therapeutic reference for major depression. Desvenlafaxine (Pristiq, **28**), the only major active renal metabolite of venlafaxine (**27**) was approved by the FDA in 2007 as the first non–hormone-based treatment for menopause. While Effexor (**27**) has an NE/5-HT affinity ratio of 30, and Pristiq (**28**) has an NE/5-HT affinity ratio of 13.8, 70% of venlafaxine (**27**) is metabolized to Pristiq (**28**), so the effects of the drugs are largely similar.[17] Milnacipran (Ixel, **29**) was approved in the United States in 2009 for the treatment of fibromyalgia but not for MDD. Although it has an NE/5-HT affinity ratio of 1.16, which is vastly different from that of venlafaxine (**27**), the two drugs are clinically equivalent in terms of efficacy, with milnacipran (Ixel, **29**) having certain advantages when sexual dysfunction, overdose, and polymedication are concerned.[18]

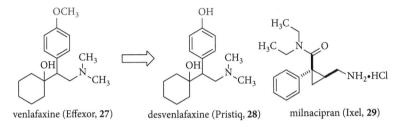

venlafaxine (Effexor, **27**)   desvenlafaxine (Pristiq, **28**)   milnacipran (Ixel, **29**)

In addition to the MAOIs, TCAs, SSRIs, and SNRIs mentioned above, other antidepressants with different MOA exist as well. For instance, Wyeth's bupropion (Wellbutrin, **30**) is a norepinephrine and dopamine reuptake inhibitors (NDRIs). It was approved in 1985 as both an atypical antidepressant and a smoking cessation aid. Trazodone (Depyrel, **31**) is a serotonin receptor antagonist and reuptake inhibitor (SARI). The drug is approved and marketed in several countries for the treatment of MDD in adult patients.[19] On the other hand, vilazodone (Viibryd, **32**) is a serotonin partial agonist and reuptake inhibitor (SPARI).[20] Lundebeck's vortioxetine (Brintellix, **33**) was approved by the FDA for the treatment of MDD in 2013. It is a novel multimodal compound for the treatment of MDD with combined effects on 5-HT3A and 5-HT1A receptors and on the serotonin transporter (SERT).[21]

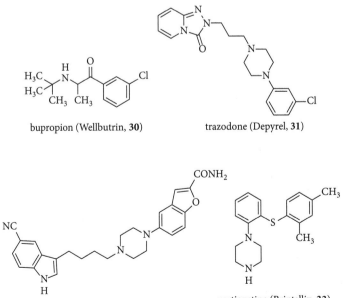

bupropion (Wellbutrin, **30**)   trazodone (Depyrel, **31**)

vilazodone (Viibryd, **32**)   vortioxetine (Brintellix, **33**)

In addition to all the dual reuptake inhibitors, serotonin–norepinephrine–dopamine reuptake inhibitors, also known as *triple reuptake inhibitors*, have been intensively studied during the last decade.[22] Although no triple reuptake inhibitors have been licensed in the US just yet, this class of antidepressants could provide better and faster onset medicine to treat MDD.

The focus of this chapter is Lilly's duloxetine hydrochloride (Cymbalta, **1**), an SNRI. It reached the market in 1994 and was a blockbuster drug, racking up to $6.3 billion in sales in 2013. It became available as a generic in December 2013.

■ 2 PHARMACOLOGY

2.1 Mechanism of Action

Cymbalta (**1**) is a dual monoamine modulator. It binds selectively with high affinity to both NE and serotonin (5-HT) transporters and lacks affinity for monoamine receptors within the central nervous system.[23–28]

In vitro, Cymbalta (**1**) inhibits both norepinephrine and serotonin uptake carriers with Ki values of 7.5nM and 0.8 nM, respectively.[23] This translates to an NE/5-HT ratio of 9.4. It does not appear to directly modulate dopaminergic function. Similar to TCAs, Cymbalta (**1**) has no affinity for dopamine transporter (DAT, Ki 240 nM) and no significant binding affinity for dopamine, serotonin, adrenergic, histaminic, or opioid receptors. It does not affect the activity of γ-aminobutyric acid (GABA) transporter and MAO activity either. So it is a relatively clean (meaning selective) drug. In vitro inhibition profiles of radioligand binding to human monoamine transporters by Cymbalta (**1**), venlafaxine (**27**), and milnacipran (**29**), also all SNRIs, are listed in Table 7.1 for comparison purposes.[24]

In rat animal models,[25] while acute administration of Cymbalta (**1**) increases both NE and 5-HT concentrations in identified rat brain regions, chronic administration of Cymabalta over 14 days does not alter basal monoamine levels in rat frontal cortex and nucleus acumens. This observation is consistent with other antidepressants.

In clinical trials, Cymbalta (**1**) inhibits binding to the human NE and 5-HT transporters with Ki values of 2.1 and 0.3 nM, respectively. In a study of healthy human volunteers receiving Cymbalta (either 20 or 60 mg/day) or placebo, Cymbalta (**1**) has a profile of a selective 5-HT reuptake inhibitor and its effect on whole blood 5-HT content confirms the serotonergic profile of this agent. Based on a considerable body

TABLE 7.1. *Transporter binding profiles of antidepressants* **1**, **27**, *and* **29**[23]

	duloxetine (**1**) Ki (nM)	venlafaxine (**27**) Ki (nM)	milnacipran (**29**) Ki (nM)
5-HT Transporter (SERT)	0.53	82	123
NE Transporter (NET)	2.1	2,480	200
DA Transporter (DAT)	240	7,647	> 10,000
NET/SERT Ratio	4	30	1.6

of evidence, Cymbalta at dosages ranging from 40 to 120 mg/day was effective in the short- and long-term treatment of MDD. Similar to most other antidepressants, onset takes approximately two to three weeks after dosing. Significant improvements versus placebo in core emotional symptoms as well as painful physical symptoms associated with depression were seen in most, but not all, appropriately designed studies.[26]

Cymbalta (**1**) is the first relatively balanced SNRI to be widely available for three indications: major depressive disorder, peripheral diabetic neuropathic pain, and female stress urinary incontinence, although it is not currently approved for all indications in all countries.

2.2 Structure–Activity Relationship

The structure–activity relationship (SAR) around compound **34** was extensively investigated.[28] Before arriving at the general structure **34**, Lilly's SAR showed that substitution of the amine side-chain was optimal with three carbons between the nitrogen and the oxygen atoms and it was preferable to have oxygen attached at the 1-position of the naphthalene in comparison to the 2-position. As far as the substituent R was concerned (see Table 7.2), substituted phenyl groups were investigated. However, introduction of electron-donating, electron-withdrawing, or neutral substituents in any of the 2-, 3-, or 4-positions of the phenyl ring did not improve the affinity of the NE transporter. Efforts on making R a heterocycle were more fruitful. As shown in Table 7.2, the thienyl analogs **1** and **36**, furan-2-yl analog **37**, and thiazolyl analog **38** demonstrated improved 5-HT uptake inhibition, with the furan analog (**37**) as the most potent serotonin reuptake inhibitor, having a Ki value of 0.7 nM.

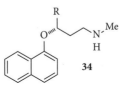

TABLE 7.2. *Binding affinities at the norepinephrine and serotonin transporters for the heterocyclic naphthyl ethers **1** and **35–38***[28]

Compound	R	5-HT	NE
35	–Ph	2.4	20
1	(thienyl, S)	1.4	20
36	(thienyl, S)	1.1	21
37	(furan, O)	0.7	20
38	(thiazolyl, N, O)	6.4	25

2.3 Bioavailability, Metabolism, and Toxicology

In animal models,[25,29] Cymbalta (**1**) is well absorbed, but extensively metabolized in rats and dogs. After single oral or intravenous 5 mg/kg doses, the absolute bioavailability is estimated to be 21% in rats and 5% in dogs. Nonetheless, studies using radiolabeled Cymbalta (**1**) show that 82% of an oral dose is absorbed in rats and 100% is absorbed in dogs.[29-33] Cymbalta (**1**) is highly bound to rat and dog plasma proteins. The mean percentage bound at a Cymbalta (**1**) concentration of 150 ng/mL is 96% in rats and 97% in dogs. Metabolism of Cymbalta (**1**) constitutes the major route of clearance in both rats and dogs followed by excretion of the metabolites into bile (feces). Cymbalta (**1**) metabolism in rats includes oxidation in the naphthyl ring, followed by further oxidation and conjugation or formation of a dihydrodiol. The major biotransformation pathway is oxidation. Urinary excretion of metabolites accounts for about 22% of a Cymbalta (**1**) dose in rats and about 29% in dogs.[29]

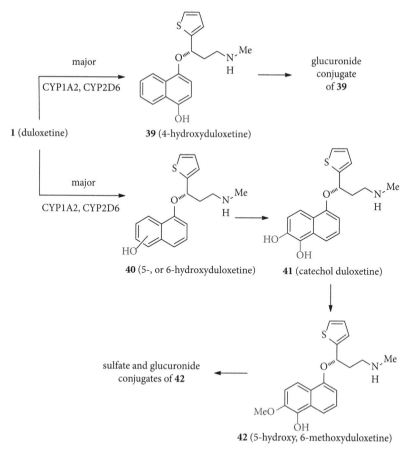

Scheme 1. Metabolism pathways and cytochrome P450 enzymes (CYPs) involved in the major oxidation steps of duloxetine biotransformation[29]

In clinical trials,[30] Cymbalta (**1**) is also highly protein-bound (95%). It achieves a C_{max} of approximately 47 ng/mL (40 mg twice-daily dosing) to 110 ng/mL (80 mg twice-daily dosing) approximately 6 h after dosing. Its elimination half-life is approximately 10–12 h and the volume of distribution is approximately 1640 L. The absolute oral bioavailability averaged 50%, ranging from 30% to 80%, after a 60 mg single dose in one study. A single dose of 60 mg Cymbalta produced a mean AUC from time zero to infinity of 591 ng•h/mL and 40 or 60 mg twice-daily dosing provided a mean steady-state AUC (AUC_{ss}) of 412 or 1050 ng•h/mL, respectively.

As far as metabolism of Cymbalta (**1**) in humans is concerned, it undergoes extensive metabolism into a complex array of metabolites (Scheme 1). Importantly, the major biotransformation pathways involve oxidation in the naphthyl ring (first-pass metabolism) followed by further oxidation, methylation, and conjugation (second-pass metabolism). The two major circulating metabolites of Cymbalta are the glucuronide conjugate of 4-hydroxy-duloxetine (**39**) and the sulfate conjugate of 5-hydroxy-6-methoxy-duloxetine (**42**). Studies were performed to determine the CYP450 enzymes responsible for the biotransformations of Cymbalta to 4-, 5-, and 6-hydroxy-duloxetine.[31] The studies correlated the formation of these metabolites with markers of CYP enzymes in a human liver microsome bank, assessed which complementary DNA (cDNA)-expressed CYPs formed the metabolites, and utilized CYP inhibitors to determine which CYP enzymes were responsible for the initial oxidation step. Because CYP450 2D6 is largely responsible for Cymbalta's (**1**) metabolism, the exposure of Cymbalta (**1**) with CYP2D6 inhibitors or in CYP2D6 poor metabolizers is increased to a lesser extent than that observed with CYP1A2 inhibition and does not require a dose adjustment. In addition, Cymbalta (**1**) increases the exposure of drugs that are metabolized by CYP2D6 but not CYP1A2.

Cymbalta's (**1**) toxicology profile is similar to that of other modern antidepressants such as SSRIs. Generally, Cymbalta (**1**) is safe and well tolerated across indications, with few reported serious side effects.[32,33] Common adverse events are consistent with the pharmacology of the molecule and are mainly referable to the gastrointestinal and the nervous systems. Treatment with Cymbalta (**1**) was associated with mild to moderate sexual dysfunction, nausea, headache, dry mouth, somnolence, and dizziness.

The studied dose range is up to 400 mg/day (administered 200 mg b.i.d [i.e., twice daily]) but the maximum dose approved for marketing is 120 mg/day (administered 60 mg b.i.d). No increase in death from suicide or in suicidal thoughts and behavior were detected as compared to placebo. So as to avoid discontinuation syndrome as a consequence of abrupt withdrawal of Cymbalta, 2 weeks of tapering is recommended before discontinuation. Overall, Cymbalta was found to be well tolerated and can be safely administered even in older patients and in those with concomitant illnesses.

■ 3 SYNTHESIS

Synthesis of Cymbalta (**1**) has been the subject of intensive efforts by many in academia and industry. Herein, only the discovery route and a typical process route are summarized.[34]

3.1 Discovery Route

The original synthesis of Cymbalta (**1**) is relatively straightforward, involving a four-step sequence from readily available 2-acetylthiophene **43** (Scheme 2).[27] A Mannich reaction of **43** with formaldehyde polymer and dimethylamine–hydrochloride salt generated β-aminoketone **44**, which was then reduced by NaBH$_4$ to provide intermediate racemic β-aminoalcohol **45** as a racemate. The desired optically active (*S*)-alcohol **45a** was accessed via resolution of racemate **45** with (*S*)-(+)-mandelic acid, which provided the necessary substrate **45a** for etherification with 1-fluoronaphthalene to afford optically active amine **46**. Finally, *N*-demethylation with 2,2,2-trichloroethyl chloroformate and cleavage of the intermediate carbamate with zinc powder and formic acid led to the desired target Cymbalta (**1**).

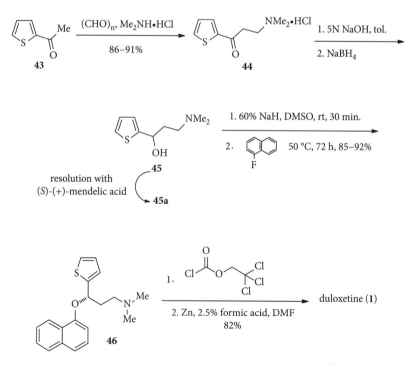

Scheme 2. Discovery route for the synthesis of duloxetine (**1**)[27]

In addition to resolution and asymmetric reduction of ketone **44** using the Yamaguchi–Masher–Pohland (YMP) complex,[36] Lilly's medicinal chemists also reported an alternative synthetic route using the Corey–Bakshi–Shibata (CBS) reagent (Scheme 3).[27] The key ketone intermediate **48** was assembled from thiophene carboxylic acid (**47**) in three steps—acid chloride formation followed by Stille coupling with tributyl(vinyl)tin and addition of hydrogen chloride across the newly formed double bond. Reduction using catalytic oxazaborolidine (*R*)-Me-CBS (**49a**) gave rise to alcohol **50a** as the *S* enantiomer. Similarly, reduction utilizing catalytic oxazaborolidine (*S*)-Me-CBS (**49b**) provided access to alcohol **50b** as the *R* enantiomer.

Now with both alcohol enantiomers **50a** and **50b** in hand, it was more straightforward to use both of them to prepare Cymbalta (**1**). An S$_N$2 reaction using NaI followed by another S$_N$2 reaction using methylamine converted **50a** to amine **51**. A subsequent S$_N$Ar reaction of the alkoxide from **51** with 1-fluoronaphthalene afforded Cymbalta (**1**). On the other hand, a Mitsunobu inversion of (*R*)-chloroalcohol **50b** was followed by iodination to provide intermediate (*S*)-ether iodide **52**, which then underwent amination to deliver the final product Cymbalta (**1**).

A synthesis of radio-labeled Cymbalta was reported by applying similar chemistry described above.[37]

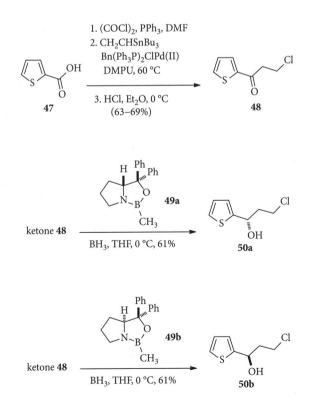

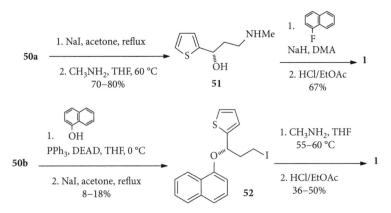

Scheme 3. Asymmetric synthesis from alcohol **50a** and **50b**[38]

3.2 Process Route

Like all blockbuster drugs, the process synthesis of Cymbalta (**1**) has been the subject of intensive efforts from both academia and industry.[38-46]

Lilly's process route involved a resolution–racemization–recycle (RRR) synthesis of Cymbalta (**1**).[38] It began with the Mannich reaction similar to the discovery route, converting aminoketone **43** to β-aminoketone **44** (Scheme 4). The HCl salt of β-aminoketone **44** was freed by base treatment and the free base was reduced by NaBH$_4$. Acidic workup was necessary to break both B–O and B–N linkages. Another round of basification afforded alcohol (±)-**45** as a racemate. To a methyl-t-butyl ether (MTBE) solution of (±)-**45** was added (S)-mandelic acid (0.45 equiv) in EtOH. The resulting slurry in MTBE/EtOH (9.8:1) was heated to reflux and then cooled to ambient temperature to allow **45a** to form a diastereomeric salt **54** with (S)-mandelic acid, during which (R)-**45b** was left unaffected and remained dissolved in the solution. The precipitated salt **53** is collected by filtration and treated with aqueous NaOH solution to liberate the desired enantiomer (S)-**45a**. In the meantime, the MTBE solution of the undesired (R)-**45b** recovered as the filtrate (mother liquor) was treated with HCl to racemize (R)-**45b** to give racemate **45** for another round of the resolution (recycling).

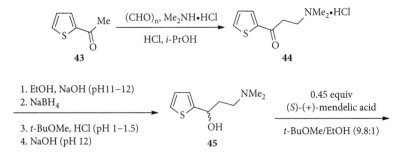

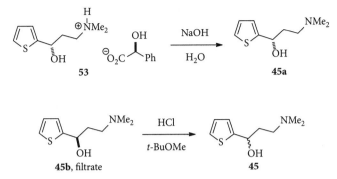

Scheme 4. Process Route for the Preparation of (S)-alcohol **45a**[38]

Taking a page from the discovery route, alcohol **45a** was treated with 1 equiv of NaH in the presence of potassium benzoate in dimethyl sulfoxide (DMSO) (Scheme 5). Addition of 1.2 equiv 1-fluoronaphthalene provided the S_NAr reaction product that was isolated as its phosphate salt **46′** of 91% *ee* in 79.6% yield. The salt was freed using ammonia and the free amine was dissolved in toluene and treated with Hünig base followed by 1.25 equiv PhOCOCl to provide *N*-demethylation product **54** at 55 °C. After alkaline hydrolysis of phenyl carbamate **54** without isolation, the aqueous workup was done by acidification to pH 5.0–5.5 with AcOH. Finally, the compound was subjected to basification to pH 10.5 with 50% aqueous NaOH solution, extraction with AcOEt followed by salt formation with HCl in the AcOEt solution eventually delivered Cymbalta (**1**) as a white solid in an overall yield of 32% from **45a**.

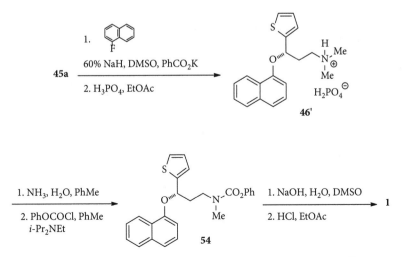

Scheme 5. Process route for the synthesis of duloxetine hydrochloride (**1**)[45]

■ 4 CONCLUDING REMARKS

In December 2013, Eli Lilly's blockbuster antidepressant Cymbalta went off patent. Cymbalta's generic version, known as duloxetine, rushes into the market and drives down the price, making it more affordable.

Great news for everyone, right?

Well, not quite.

Indeed, generic competition is a great boon to the payer and the patient. On the other hand, the makers of the brand medicines can lose about 70% of the revenue. Without sustained investment in drug discovery and development, there will be fewer and fewer lifesaving drugs, not really a scenario the patient wants. Cymbalta had sales of $6.3 billion in 2013. Combined with Zyprexa, which lost patent protection in 2011, Lilly lost $10 billion in annual sales from these two drugs alone. The company responded by freezing salaries and slashing 30% of its sales force.

Lilly is not alone in this quandary. In 2011, Pfizer lost patent protection for its $13 billion drug Lipitor, the best-selling drug ever, which made "merely" $2.3 billion in 2013. Of course Pfizer became the number one drug company by swallowing Warner-Lambert, Pharmacia, and Wyeth, shutting down many research sites that were synonyms to the American pharmaceutical industry and shedding tens of thousands of jobs. Meanwhile, Merck lost US marketing exclusivity of its asthma drug Singulair (montekulast) in 2012 and saw a 97% decline in US sales in the fourth quarter of 2012 compared with the fourth quarter of 2011. Merck announced in October 2013 that it would cut 8,500 jobs on top of the 7,500 layoffs planned earlier. Peak sales of BMS's Plavix (clopidogrel) were $7 billion, making it the second-best-selling drug ever. After Plavix lost its patent protection in May 2012, the sales were $258 million in 2013. Meanwhile BMS has shrunk from 43,000 to 28,000 employees in the last decade.

Generic competition is not the only woe that Big Pharma is facing. Outsourcing pharma jobs to China and India, merger and acquisition (M&A), and the economic downturn forced thousands of highly paid and highly educated scientists to scramble for alternative employments, many outside the drug industry. With numerous site closures, outsourcing cost reductions, and downsizing, some 150,000 in Big Pharma lost their jobs from 2009 through 2012, according to consulting firm Challenger, Gray & Christmas. Such a brain drain makes us the lost generation of American drug discovery scientists. In contrast, Japanese drug companies refused to improve the bottom line through mass layoffs of R&D staff, a decision that will likely benefit productivity in the long run.

What can we do to ensure the health of the drug industry and sustain the output of lifesaving medicines? Realizing that there is no single prescription for this issue, one could certainly begin by talking about patent reform.

The current patent system is antiquated as far as innovative drugs are concerned. Decades ago, 17 years of patent life was adequate time for the drug companies to recoup their investment in R&D because the lifecycle from discovery to marketing at the time was relatively short and the cost was lower. Today's drug discovery and development is a completely new ballgame. First of all, the low-hanging fruits have been harvested and it is becoming increasingly challenging to create novel drugs, especially those that are "first-in-class" medicines. Second, the clinical trials are longer and use more patients, increasing the cost and eating into patent life. The latest statistics say that it takes $1.3 billion to take a drug from idea to market after taking the failed drugs' costs into account. This is the major reason why prescription drugs are so expensive—pharmaceutical companies need to recoup their investment so that they will have money to invest in discovering future lifesaving medicines. Today's patent life of 20 years (patent life was extended in 1995) is insufficient, especially for those drugs that are "first-in-class."

Therefore, patent life for innovative medicines should be extended, because the risk is the highest, as is the failure rate. Since the lifecycle from idea to regulatory approval is getting longer and longer, it would make more sense if the patent clock started ticking after the drug is approved and exclusivity is still provided after the filing.

Top executives are receiving millions of dollars in compensation even as the company is laying off thousands of employees to reduce cost. The current compensation system for the discovery of lifesaving drugs is in a dire need of reform as well. The situation is beginning to change. Recently, for example, GlaxoSmithKline announced that the company will pay significant bonuses to scientists who discover drugs. This is a good start.

The phenomenon of blockbuster drugs was a harbinger of the golden age of the pharmaceutical industry. Patients were happy because taking medicines was vastly cheaper than staying in the hospital. Shareholders were happy because huge profits were made and stocks for Big Pharma used to be considered a sure bet. Perhaps most importantly, the drug industry expanded and employed more and more scientists and engineers in its workforce. That employment in turn encouraged academia to train more students in science. America's science, technology, engineering, and mathematics (STEM) education was and still is the envy of the rest of the world. Maintaining that important reputation depends on a thriving pharmaceutical industry to provide jobs for our leading scientists and researchers. In turn they will reward us by discovering the next life-saving drugs.

■ 5 REFERENCES

1. Ayd, F. J. Jr.; Blackwell, B., Eds. *Discoveries in the Biological Psychiatry*. J. B. Lippincott Co.: Philadelphia, 1970.

2. Bosworth, D. M. *Ann. New York Acad. Sci.* **1959**, *80*, 809–819.

3. Davis, W. A. *J. Clin. Exp. Psychopath.* **1958**, *19 (Suppl. 1)*, 1–10.

4. Kauffman, G. B. *J. Chem. Ed.* **1979**, *56*, 35–36.

5. Kamada, T.; Chow, T.; Hiroi, T.; Imaoka, S.; Morimoto, K.; Ohde, H.; Funae, Y. *Drug Metab. Dispos.* **2002**, *17*, 199–206.

6. Shin, H.-S. *Drug Metab. Dispos.* **1997**, *25*, 657–662.

7. Laux, G.; Volz, H.-P.; Moeller, H.-J. *CNS Drugs* **1995**, *3*, 145–158.

8. Kuhn, A. *Am. J. Psychiatry* **1958**, *115*, 459–464.

9. Evrard, D. A.; Harrison, B. L. *Ann. Rep. Med. Chem.* **1999**, *34*, 1–9.

10. Feighner, J. P. *J. Clin. Psychiatry*, **1999**, *60 (Suppl 22)*, 18–22.

11. Spinks, D.; Spinks, G. *Curr. Med. Chem.* **2002**, *9*, 799–810.

12. Sussman, N. *J. Clin. Psychiatry* **2003**, *5 (Suppl. 7)*, 19–26.

13. Gillman, P. K. *Br. J. Pharmacol.* **2007**, *151*, 737–748.

14. Wenthur, C. J.; Bennett, M. R.; Lindsley, C. W. *Bioorg. Med. Chem. Lett.* **2014**, *5*, 14–23.

15. Hopkins, C. R. *ACS Chem. Neurosci.* **2011**, *2*, 554–554.

16. Lee, Y.-C.; Chen, P.-P. *Expert Opin. Pharmacother.* **2010**, *11*, 2813–2825.

17. Dell'Osso, B.; Buoli, M.; Baldwin, D. S.; Altamura, A. C. *Hum. Psychopharmacol. Clin. Exp.* **2010**, *25*, 17–29.

18. Mansuy, L. *Neuropsychiatric Disease Treat.* **2010**, *6 (Suppl I)*, 17–22.

19. Fagiolini, A.; Comandini, A.; Dell'Osso, M. C.; Kasper, S. *CNS Drugs* **2012**, *26*, 1033–1049.

20. Schwartz, T. L.; Siddiqui, U. A.; Stahl, S. M. *Ther. Adv. Psychopharmacol.* **2011**, *1*, 81–87.

21. Bang-Andersen, B.; Ruhland, T.; Jørgensen, M. et al. *J. Med. Chem.* **2011**, *54*, 3206–3221.

22. Chen, Z.; Skolnick, P. *Expert Opin. Invest. Drugs* **2007**, *16*, 1365–1377.

23. Karpa, K. D.; Cavanaugh, J. E.; Lakoski, J. M. *CNS Drug Rev.* **2002**, *8*, 361–376.

24. Stahl, S. M.; Grady, M. M; Moret, C.; Briley, M. *CNS Spectrums* **2005**, *10*, 732–747.

25. Torres-Sanchez, S.; Perez-Caballero, L.; Mico, J. A.; Elorza, J.; Berrocoso, E. *Expert Opin. Drug Discov.* **2012**, *7*, 745–755.

26. Frampton, J. E.; Plosker, G. L. *CNS Drugs* **2007**, *21*, 581–609.

27. Bymaster, F. P.; Beedle, E. E.; Findlay, J.; Gallagher, P. T.; Krushinski, J. H.; Mitchell, S.; Robertson, D. W.; Thompson, D. C.; Wallace, L.; Wong, D. T. *Bioorg. Med. Chem. Lett.* **2003**, *13*, 4477–4480.

28. Bymaster, F. P.; Lee, T. C.; Knadler, M. P.; Detke, M. J.; Iyengar, S. *Current Pharmaceutical Design* **2005**, *11*, 1475–1493.

29. Knadler, M. P.; Lobo, E.; Chappell, J.; Bergstrom, R. *Clin. Pharmacokinetics* **2011**, *50*, 281–294.

30. Lantz, R. J.; Gillespie, T. A.; Rash, T. J. et al. *Drug Metab. Dispos.* **2003**, *31*, 1142–1150.

31. Kuo, F.; Gillespie, T. A.; Kulanthaivel, P.; Lantz, R. J.; Ma, T. W.; Nelson, D. L.; Threlkeld, P. G.; Wheeler, W. J.; Yi, P.; Zmijewski, M. *Bioorg. Med. Chem. Lett.* **2004**, *14*, 3481–3486.

32. Wernicke, J. F.; Gahimer, J.; Yalcin, I.; Wulster-Radcliffe, M.; Viktrup, L. *Exp. Opin. Drug Safety* **2005**, *4*, 987–993.

33. Bitter, I.; Filipovits, D.; Czobor, P. *Exp. Opin. Drug Safety* **2011**, *10*, 839–850.

34. Pineiro-Nunez, M. Advances in development of methods for the synthesis of dual selective serotonin and norepinephrine reuptake inhibitors (SSNRIs) [venlafaxine hydrochloride (Effexor), milnacipran hydrochloride (Ixel, Dalcipran) and duloxetine hydrochloride (Cymbalta)], in *Art of Drug Synthesis*, Johnson, D. S.; Li, J. J., Eds.; Wiley: Hoboken, NJ, 2007, pp. 199–213.

35. Robertson, D.; Wong, D.; Krushinski, J. US Patent 5023269 (1991).

36. Deeter, J.; Frazier, J; Staten, G.; Staszak, M.; Weigel, L. *Tetrahedron Lett.* **1990**, *31*, 7101–7104.

37. Wheeler, W.; Kuo, F. *J. Label. Compd. Radiopharm.* **1995**, *36*, 213–223.

38. Berglund, R. US Patent 5362886 (1994).

39. Borghese, A. WO 062219 (2003).

40. Liu, H.; Hoff, B. H.; Anthonsen, T. *Chirality* **2000**, *12*, 26–29.

41. Kamal, A.; Ramesh Khanna, G. B.; Ramu, R.; Krishnaji, T. *Tetrahedron Lett.* **2003**, *44*, 4783–4787.

42. Noyori, R.; Koizumi, M.; Ishii, D.; Ohkuma, T. *Pure Appl. Chem.* **2001**, *73*, 227–232.

43. Ratovelomanana-Vidal, V.; Girard, C.; Touati, R.; Tranchier, J. P.; Ben Hassine, B.; Genêt, J. P. *Adv. Synth. Catal.* **2003**, *345*, 261–274.

44. Liu, D.; Gao, W.; Wang, C.; Zhang, X. *Angew. Chem. Int. Ed.* **2005**, *44*, 1687–1689.

45. Fujima, Y; Ikunaka, M; Inoue, T; Matsumoto, J. *Org. Process Res. Dev.* **2006**, *10*, 905–913.

46. Astleford, B. A.; Weigel, L. O. Resolution versus stereoselective synthesis in drug development: some case studies, in *Chirality in Industry II: Developments in the Commercial Manufacture and Applications of Optically Active Compounds*; Collins, A. N., Sheldrake, G. N., Crosby, J., Eds.; Wiley: Chichester, UK, 1997; pp. 99–117.

8   Olanzapine (Zyprexa)

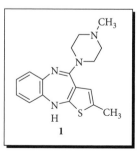

1

USAN:	*Olanzapine*
Brand Name:	*Zyprexa (Eli Lilly)*
Molecular Weight:	*312.43*
FDA Approval:	*1996*
Drug Class:	*Atypical Antipsychotic Drug*
Indications:	*Schizophrenia and Bipolar Disorder*
Mechanism of Action:	*Serotonin–Dopamine Antagonist (SDA)*

■ 1 HISTORY OF SCHIZOPHRENIA AND ANTIPSYCHOTIC DRUGS

Schizophrenia is a devastating mental disorder, inflicting 1.1% of the population over the age of 18, which translates to 51 million people worldwide including 2.2 million people in the United States. Schizophrenia strikes men and women at different ages; the average onset age is 18 for men and 25 for women.

Schizophrenia is characterized by *positive symptoms* such as delusions, hallucinations, and disorganized speech/behavior and *negative symptoms* including apathy, withdrawal, lack of pleasure, and impaired attention.[1] While it might be relatively easy to treat positive symptoms with antipsychotics, negative symptoms are more difficult to treat. Other symptoms include depressive/anxious symptoms and aggressive symptoms such as hostility, verbal and physical abusiveness, and impulsivity. Because of schizophrenia's complexity, it is challenging to find therapeutics that are both efficacious and safe, especially considering that the patient has to take them for a prolonged period of time.[2]

In ancient times, an "insane" person was often thought to be possessed by the devil, or he was being punished by God for his sins. As a consequence, beating, bleeding, starvation, hot- and cold-water shock treatment, restraint, and incarceration were widely practiced on mental patients, which only worsened their conditions.

In 1927, Austrian neurologist Julius Wagner von Jauregg invented the fever shock treatment, introducing malaria in psychotics. Egaz Moniz invented the lobotomy to "introduce an organic syndrome" for the treatment of schizophrenia; both men won the Nobel Prize (for Physiology or Medicine). Today, neither malaria introduction nor lobotomy is still in use.[3]

Although there is still a certain stigma attached to mental illnesses, we have now amassed a tremendous amount of knowledge with regard to the genetic, biochemical, and environmental impacts on the human brain. Psychopharmacological drugs such as olanzapine (Zyprexa, **1**) have significantly contributed to managing and understanding mental diseases including schizophrenia.

1.1 Typical Antipsychotics—The First Generation

Before chlorpromazine (**2**) became available in 1962, early treatments for schizophrenia included prolonged narcosis, known as "narcosis for psychosis." Meanwhile, history also saw the use of excruciating treatments such as electroshock and shock introduced by fever, methiazole, and insulin. Older CNS drugs such as opiates, belladonna derivatives, bromides, barbiturates, antihistamines, and chloral hydrates (each with its unique efficacy and safety profile) have all been used to treat schizophrenia with different degrees of "success."

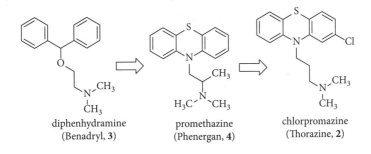

diphenhydramine
(Benadryl, **3**)

promethazine
(Phenergan, **4**)

chlorpromazine
(Thorazine, **2**)

The genesis of chlorpromazine (**2**) can be traced back to antihistamines. In 1944, a group of scientists at Rhône-Poulenc Laboratories, led by chemist Paul Charpentier, began a program to systematically search for safer antihistamines. Their starting point was older antihistamines such as diphenhydramines (Benadryl, **3**). In time, they successfully synthesized and marketed the antihistamine promethazine (Phenergan, **4**). Similar to most antihistamines, promethazine (**4**) had side effects in the CNS that included mild antipsychotic properties. Charpentier sought to enhance these "side effects." Structural–activity relationship (SAR) investigations led to the synthesis of RP-3277 (chlorpromazine, **2**) in 1950.[4] It was tested in rats, which became "indifferent." In clinical trials, patients, too, became "disinterested" under the influence of chlorpromazine (**2**). In addition to the outstanding "calming" activities of RP-3277, it was later determined to have low toxicity. More importantly, chlorpromazine (**2**) subdued the positive symptoms (such

as hallucinations and delusions) of psychotic patients.[5] Chlorpromazine was introduced in 1952 in France under the trade name Largactil. The Largactil (meaning
large activity) was chosen to reflect the wide range of CNS activities that chlorpromazine elicited. It was the first conventional (typical) antipsychotic discovered
that was superior to opium. Chlorpromazine (**2**) was introduced to the US in 1954
under the trade name Thorazine. In the first eight months, the drug was administered to more than two million patients. It contributed to an 80% reduction of the
resident population in mental hospitals. Thorazine (**2**) added a great impetus to
the beginning of the psychopharmacological revolution.

Subsequently, Thorazine (**2**) was shown to be a potent dopamine D_2 antagonist
with other pharmacological properties that were thought to cause unwanted side
effects. Thus, the D_2-receptor antagonism of the conventional antipsychotics is
thought to be responsible not only for their therapeutic effects, but also for some
of their side effects. In addition, Thorazine (**2**) also helped our understanding of
the CNS through research into the drug's MOA.

Many "me-too" (copy-cat) drugs emerged soon after Thorazine's (**2**) success.[6] They
included fluphenazine (Sinqualone, **5**), perphenazine (Trilafon, **6**), trifluoperazine
(Stelazine, **7**), and thioridazine (Melleril, **8**). Incidentally, fluphenazine (**5**), along with
5-fluorouracil, was one of the first fluorine-containing drugs. Collectively known as
typical antipsychotics, they all belong to the phenothiazine class. Unfortunately, they
all cause a common group of side effects known as extrapyramidal symptoms (EPS),
which Parkinsonian symptoms, akathisia, dyskinesia, and dystonia.

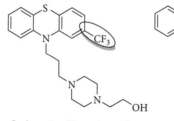
fluphenazine (Sinqualone, **5**)

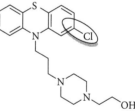
perphenazine (Trilafon, **6**)

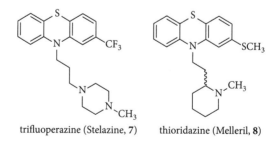
trifluoperazine (Stelazine, **7**)　　thioridazine (Melleril, **8**)

Another typical antipsychotic, haloperidol (Haldol, **9**), is *not* a phenothiazine.
Before the emergence of atypical antipsychotics, it was the gold standard for treating schizophrenia. Prepared in 1958 in Paul Janssen's laboratories and distinctive

from chlorpromazine (2) and other phenothiazines, Haldol (9) was a butyrophenone derivative. Therefore, Haldol's chlorpromazine-like activity came as a surprise to Janssen and his colleagues. Haldol (9) was both faster and longer acting; it was potent orally as well as parentally; and more importantly, it was almost devoid of the anti-adrenergic and other autonomic effects associated with chlorpromazine (2). Haldol (9) also had a more favorable safety ratio and was surprisingly well tolerated when given chronically to laboratory animals.

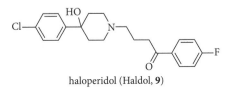

haloperidol (Haldol, 9)

Clinical trials confirmed that Haldol (9) belonged to the pharmacological family of neuroleptics. It became valuable in the treatment of agitation, delusions, and hallucinations in mental patients. Numerous chronic inpatients were able to leave the hospital and live at home thanks to Haldol (9). Until the emergence of atypical antipsychotics, Haldol remained one of the more prescribed neuroleptics 40 years after its discovery.

Haldol (9) was 50–100 times more potent than Thorazine (2), with fewer side effects—it was the most potent antipsychotic at the time of its discovery. It was developed as a more potent and selective D_2 antagonist because the D_2-receptor blockade in the mesolimbic pathway is believed to reduce the positive symptoms of schizophrenia. Indeed, Haldol (9) is very effective against the positive systems, however, like all other typical antipsychotics, it is ineffective in treating the negative symptoms and neurocognitive deficits of schizophrenia. In addition, administration of the drug typically causes EPS similar to other typical antipsychotics.[7]

With the discovery of newer atypical antipsychotics, older conventional antipsychotics are no longer used as first-line therapy, but can still be effective as a second-line or add-on treatment.

1.2 Atypical Antipsychotics—The Second Generation

As mentioned in the previous section, Haldol (9) and other typical antipsychotics are efficacious in treating positive symptoms of schizophrenia. But they are ineffective in treating the negative symptoms and neurocognitive deficits of schizophrenia. In addition, administration of typical antipsychotics often causes EPS.[8]

Clozapine (Clozaril, 10), the first atypical antipsychotic, was developed in 1959 by a small Swiss company, Wander AG.[9] During clinical trials, Clozaril (10) showed strong sedating effects and proved efficacious for schizophrenia, but also showed some liver toxicity. Wander planned to withdraw the drug because of expected difficulty receiving regulatory approval, but clinicians who conducted trials urged

Wander to provide more samples because their patients fared better on Clozaril (10) than on typical antipsychotics. For a population of patients who responded poorly to standard therapy at the time, Clozaril (10) was especially effective. Wander AG reluctantly proceeded with more trials of Clozaril and received approval to market it in a few European countries in 1971—although liver toxicity limited its widespread use. Unfortunately, the drug was eventually removed from the market in 1975 due to drug-associated agranulocytosis, a rare but potentially fatal blood disorder that resulted in lowered white-cell counts, which occurred in approximately 2–3% of patients. In Finland, eight patients died from subsequent infections. Additional side effects of Clozaril (10) therapy include sedation, weight gain, and orthostatic hypotension. Clozaril (10) was reintroduced in 1990 by Sandoz, and is now used as a second-line treatment—extensive monitoring of the patient's blood cell count is required. Over the years Clozaril has demonstrated efficacy against treatment-resistant schizophrenia and some still consider it the gold standard treatment for refractory patients despite the inconvenience of a weekly check of white blood cell counts.

Clozaril (10) is considered the first atypical antipsychotic. Atypical antipsychotics, sometimes called serotonin–dopamine antagonists (SDAs), have reduced EPS compared to typical antipsychotics and are also believed to reduce negative, cognitive, and affective symptoms of schizophrenia more effectively. All atypical antipsychotics are potent antagonists of serotonin 5-HT$_{2A}$ and dopamine D$_2$ receptors, however they also act on many other receptors including multiple serotonin receptors (5-HT$_{1A}$, 5-HT$_{1B/1D}$, 5-HT$_{2C}$, 5-HT$_3$, 5-HT$_6$, 5-HT$_7$), the noradrenergic system (α_1 and α_2), the cholinergic system (M$_1$) and the histamine receptors (H$_1$).

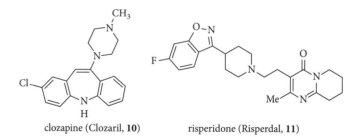

clozapine (Clozaril, 10)   risperidone (Risperdal, 11)

The second atypical antipsychotic was risperidone (Risperdal, 11) introduced by Janssen Pharmaceuticals in Belgium in 1993. With the success of Haldol (9) on the market, Janssen systematically explored its clinical utilities. They ultimately discovered Risperdal (11). Within a series of benzisoxazole derivatives, Risperdal showed a desired combination of very potent serotonin and potent dopamine antagonism. In essence, Risperdal (11) possessed the attributes of both ritanserin (a serotonin 5HT$_2$ antagonist) and haloperidol (a dopamine antagonist), a typical antipsychotic. In schizophrenic patients, Risperdal (11) is effective against both positive and negative symptoms with reduced EPS liability and has become a first-line therapy.

The third atypical antipsychotic was Eli Lilly's Zyprexa (**1**), launched in 1996. It is an antagonist against several receptors including dopamine, serotonin, histamine, adrenergic and muscarinic receptors. It was selected from a large series of chemical analogs based on behavioral tests (see below). Like many atypical antipsychotics, one of the side effects of Zyprexa is weight gain. Ironically, the weight gain side effect of some atypical anti-psychotics may be used to advantage by being prescribed off-label to patients with anorexia.

Since 2003, Zyprexa (**1**) has consistently had revenues of over $4 billion annually. It brought in over $5 billion, or nearly 22% of Lilly's full-year sales, in 2011. The drug, which went generic in 2012, is the focus of this chapter.

Additional atypical antipsychotics include AstraZeneca's quetiapine fumarate (Seroquel, **12**, 1997), Pfizer's ziprasidone (Geodon, **13**, 2001), and BMS/Otsuka's aripiprazole (Abilify, **14**). One of the great advantages of ziprasidone (**13**) and aripiprazole (**14**) is that they do not have the weight gain side effect associated with other antipsychotics. Two more atypical antipsychotics—zotepine (Zoleptil, **15**) and sertindole (Serlect, **16**)—are available in some countries, but not in the US.

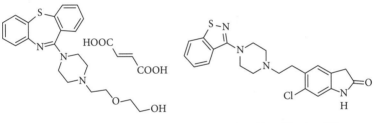

quetiapine fumarate (Seroquel, **12**)   ziprasidone (Geodon, **13**)

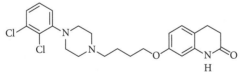

aripiprazole (Abilify, **14**)

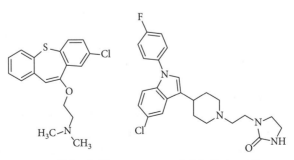

zotepine (Zoleptil, **15**)   sertindole (Serlect, **16**)

Risperdal (**11**), Zyprexa (**1**), quetiapine (**12**), ziprasidone (**13**), and aripiprazole (**14**) are currently considered as the first-line therapeutics for psychosis and will be highlighted in detail. Each of these drugs has a unique pharmacological and clinical profile; the clinician must therefore balance the benefit-risk factors for each patient in determining which drug to prescribe.[10–12]

Among the five first-line atypical antipsychotics,[13,14] Risperdal (**11**) has high affinity for D_2, 5-HT_{2C} and α_1 receptors and a very high affinity for the 5-HT_{2A} receptor, whereas quetiapine (**12**) has the lowest affinity for the D_2 and 5-HT_{2A} receptors among the atypicals, and therefore relatively high doses are required for maximal efficacy. Ziprasidone (**13**) has high affinity for the D_2 receptor, but even higher affinity for 5-HT_{2A} and 5-HT_{2C} receptors. Unlike other atypical antipsychotics, ziprasidone (**13**) also has potent 5-$HT_{1B/1D}$ antagonist and 5-HT_{1A} partial agonist activity, as well as moderate SRI/NRI activity. On the other hand, aripiprazole (**14**) is a D_2 partial agonist with an intrinsic activity of approximately 30%. Therefore, it acts as an agonist on presynaptic autoreceptors, which have a high receptor reserve, and as an antagonist on D_2 post-synaptic receptors, where significant levels of endogenous dopamine exist and there is no receptor reserve.

Much remains to be discovered about the underlying pathophysiology of schizophrenia and there is still a great need for medicinal chemists to develop more efficacious and safer drugs that are devoid of clinically limiting side-effects and also address the cognitive impairment symptoms.

■ 2 PHARMACOLOGY

2.1 Mechanism of Action

After examining 17 atypical antipsychotics, Meltzer proposed the serotonin–dopamine hypothesis in 1989.[15,16] Accordingly, atypical antipsychotic drugs may share common features such as relatively greater 5-HT_{2A} receptor binding potency than D_2 receptor binding potency. The difference between 5-HT_{2A} pKi and D_2 pKi is approximately greater than one. That is more than 10 times greater affinity for 5-HT_{2A} than for D_2 receptors. Of course only one factor, such as high 5-HT_{2A} receptor binding potency or low D_2 receptor binding potency, is not a sufficient condition. This pharmacological profile of atypical antipsychotic drugs has been thought to provide strong evidence for the serotonin–dopamine hypothesis that postulates a major contribution of the 5-HT_{2A}/D_2 receptor interactions to the MOA of these drugs.

As shown in Table 8.1, Zyprexa (**1**) is similar to all other atypical antipsychotics whose difference between 5-HT_{2A} pKi and D_2 pKi is approximately greater than one. This difference again translates to 10 times greater affinity for 5-HT_{2A} than for D_2 receptors. The only exception to the group is aripiprazole (**14**), whose affinity for 5-HT_{2A} receptor is 10 times smaller than for the D_2 receptor. More important, aripiprazole (**14**) is a partial agonist to D_2 receptors ($Ki = 0.74$). In terms of clinical ramifications, binding to D_2 receptors is associated with the drugs' antipsychotic

TABLE 8.1. *Binding potencies of atypical antipsychotics to 5HT$_{2A}$ and D$_2$ receptors*[15]

Atypical Antipsychotics	pKi, 5HT$_{2A}$	pKi, D$_2$	5HT$_{2A}$ – D$_2$
Clozapine (**10**)	8.3	7.0	1.3
Risperidone (**11**)	10.1	8.9	1.2
Olanzapine (**1**)	8.7	7.8	0.9
Quetiapine (**12**)	6.8	5.9	0.9
Ziprasidone (**13**)	9.5	8.0	1.5
Aripiprazole (**14**)	8.1	9.1	–1.0
Zotepine (**15**)	9.0	7.9	1.1

effects and EPS. On the other hand, binding to 5-HT$_{2A}$ receptors is responsible for the anti-EPS effects.[17]

Another theory also exists to explain atypical antipsychotics' MOA, which is the "fast-off" theory. In 2001, Kapur and Seeman[18] advanced a new hypothesis, which argues that fast dissociation from the dopamine D$_2$ receptor alone may explain the action of atypical antipsychotics. They argue that the difference between typical and atypical antipsychotic drugs may be fully explained by the pharmacokinetics of their interaction with the D$_2$ receptor. This fast-off theory has become an antithesis to the serotonin–dopamine hypothesis. It implies that the atypical antipsychotic effect can be produced by appropriate modulation of the D$_2$ receptor alone, while the blockade of the 5-HT$_{2A}$ receptor and other receptors may be neither necessary nor sufficient. The atypical action of clozapine (**10**) has therefore been attributed to the binding property to the D$_2$ receptor alone, but not the additional interaction with 5-HT$_{2A}$ receptors.

A couple of years later, Meltzer[19] suggested that the fast-off theory could only apply to clozapine (**10**) and quetiapine (**12**) but would not account for the pharmacological basis of other atypical antipsychotics including Zyprexa (**1**), Risperdal (**11**) and ziprasidone (**13**).

Secondary literature[20–23] that summarize the MOA and pharmacology of atypical antipsychotics is available.

2.2 Structure–Activity Relationship

Historically, Zyprexa (**1**) series evolved from clothiapine (**17**) and octoclothepin (**18**).[24–26] Both **17** and **18** are dibenzoepines and powerful typical antipsychotics. Medicinal chemists at Lilly initially intended to replace one of the benzene rings on dibenzoepines with a heterocycle and create an electronic imbalance between the two rings. Back in 1980, our understanding of antipsychotics was not as sophisticated as it is today. Lilly chemists explored their SAR using in vivo models—namely, the gross CNS activity of their compounds was established by studying the effects on the behavior of mice. Neuroleptic activity was evaluated in terms of the ability of mice to produce hypothermia in mice and to block a conditioned avoidance response and produce catalepsy in rats. They were compared with various types of antipsychotic drugs, such as Thorazine (**2**), Haldol (**9**), and Clozaril (**10**).

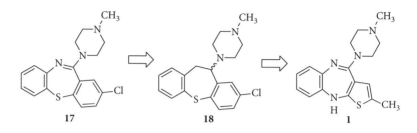

If the project were carried out today, invariably a battery of in vitro binding assays would be done for receptors including 5-HT$_{2A}$, 5-HT$_{2C}$, D$_1$, D$_2$, and D$_4$.

With respect to neuroleptic activity, it was evident from Lilly's initial SAR investigations that a basic piperazine ring attached to the thienobenzodiazepine ring at position 4 was essential. The presence of a distal nitrogen with respect to the tricyclic system also seems critical since compounds which are similarly substituted with a piperidine or morpholine ring, where this nitrogen is absent, are less effective. Compounds substituted with aminoalkylamines, where the conformational freedom of these chains is greater than that of the piperazine ring, are also less effective. This suggests that a certain conformational state of the distal nitrogen atom of the piperazine ring is required for neuroleptic activity.

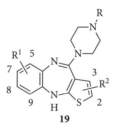

An abridged SAR table around Zyprexa (**1**) is shown in Table 8.2 where in vivo data for rat catalepsy (PO) is omitted for clarity.[24] In terms of the alkyl group R on the piperazine group (entries 1–4), 4′-(N-methylpiperazinyl) compounds are most active. Higher alkyl (Et, n-Pr) leads to a reduction in activity. When additional alcohols, amines, or carbamates are attached to N (not shown in Table 8.2), the potency is even lower. The N-oxide of the nitrogen directly attached to R is inactive, an observation seen for other antipsychotic drugs as well.

For substituents R^1 on the benzene ring on the left, 7-F- (entry 2), 7-Cl- (entry 5), and 7,8-difluoro- (entry 6) analogs seem to impart good potency although the 6,8-difluoro-analog (entry 7) shows diminished activity.

As shown in entries 8–11, a short alkyl substitution R^2 (Me, Et, i-Pr) at position 2 of the thiophene ring increased the activity. Compounds with a bulky t-Bu group (entry 10) or a long n-hexane chain (entry 11) at this position, or with 3-methyl or 2,3-dialkyl substituents, showed only minimal activity.

TABLE 8.2. *An abridged SAR table around olanzapine (1)*[24]

Entry	Compound	R	R^1	R^2	Mouse hypothermia ED_{min}, mg/kg, PO
1	**19a**	H	7-F	2-C_2H_5	100
2	**19b**	CH_3	7-F	2-C_2H_5	6.25
3	**19c**	C_2H_5	H	2-C_2H_5	50
4	**19d**	n-C_3H_7	7-F	2-C_2H_5	6.25
5	**19e**	CH_3	7-Cl	2-C_2H_5	6.25
6	**19f**	CH_3	7,8-F_2	2-C_2H_5	6.25
7	**19g**	CH_3	6,8-F	2-C_2H_5	25
8	**19h**	CH_3	7-F	CH_3	3
9	**19i**	CH_3	7-F	i-Pr	6.25
10	**19j**	CH_3	7-F	2-t-Bu	12.5
11	**19k**	CH_3	7-F	n-C_6H_{13}	100
12	chlorpromazine (**2**)				50
13	haloperidol (**9**)				3.00
14	clozapine (**10**)				6.25

2.3 Bioavailability, Metabolism, and Toxicology

Zyprexa (**1**) is well absorbed (>65%) from the gastrointestinal tract and reaches C_{max} in 6 h after oral dose.[27–31] It undergoes significant first-pass metabolism (such as oxidation, reduction, and hydrolysis), which functionalizes the drug. Second-pass metabolism refers to conjugation reactions such as sulfation and glucuronidation. For Zyprexa (**1**), approximately 40% of the dose is metabolized before reaching the system circulation.[28,29]

The volume of distribution (V_d) for human is large for Zyprexa (**1**): 22 L/kg. A range of 5–100 L/kg for V_d for man is considered high, whereas a range of 0.6–5 L/kg is considered moderate. Since the larger the V_d, the longer half-life, Zyprexa (**1**) has a half-life of 30 h. At typical plasma concentrations, it is 93% protein bound, primarily to albumin and α_1-acid glycoprotein.[28]

Zyprexa (**1**) is extensively metabolized. The major circulating metabolite of Zyprexa (**1**) is 10-*N*-glucuronide conjugate **20**, which is present at a concentration of 44% of the parent compound (see Fig. 8.1). This major metabolite is eliminated into the urine and feces where it accounts for 13% and 12% of the administered dose, respectively. The *N*-desmethyl metabolite **21** plasma concentration reaches 31% of that of Zyprexa (**1**). Both 20 and 21 are believed to be biologically inactive at these concentrations. Other identified metabolites include 4′-*N*-glucuronide **22**, *N*-oxide **23**, 2-hydroxymethyl **24**, and 2-carboxy **25**. Another metabolite is the *N*-desmethyl metabolite from 2-carboxy **25**.[26]

The mean apparent plasma clearance (CL) is 25 L/h, which is very high. In humans, apparent plasma clearance of 15–20 L/h is considered high and a clearance of 2–15 L/h is considered moderate.[29]

In terms of safety, Zyprexa (**1**) produced significantly fewer EPS such as dystonia, Parkinsonism, and akathisia than typical antipsychotics such as Haldol (**9**)[30] Unfortunately, like many atypical antipsychotics, Zyprexa (**1**) has been associated

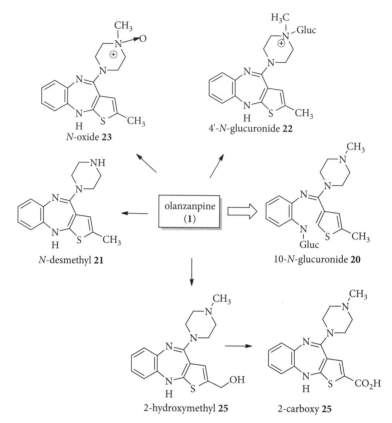

Fig. 8.1. Metabolic pathways of olanzapine (**1**) in humans[28]

with significant weight gain. The mean weight gain was 2–3 kg during the first 6 weeks of acute therapy. This is significantly greater than placebo.[31] The weight gain is probably the most detrimental side effect for Zyprexa (**1**) because weight gain is often associated with diabetes and a slew of other diseases.

▪ 3 SYNTHESIS

3.1 Discovery Route

In 1980, Chakrabarti and coworkers at Eli Lilly reported the initial discovery and synthesis of Zyprexa (**1**, Scheme 1).[24,32–37] Applying a methodology that they published in 1978,[32] they assembled the thiophene ring using a Gewald aminothiophene synthesis. Thus thiophene **26** was synthesized by adding a DMF solution of malononitrile to a mixture of sulfur, propionaldehyde and triethylamine in DMF. The anion of amino thiophene **26** after treatment with NaH underwent a nucleophilic aromatic substitution with 2-fluoronitrobenzene to provide adduct **27**. The nitro group was reduced with stannous chloride and the resulting aniline cyclized with the cyano group to form amidine **28**. Finally, a mixture of *N*-methylpipera-zine and **28** were refluxed in DMSO/toluene to deliver Zyprexa (**1**).

This synthetic route was used to synthesize the putative metabolites of Zyprexa (**1**) as well.[26]

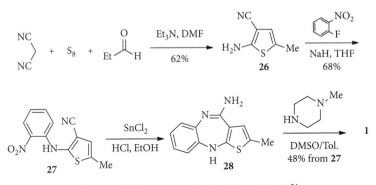

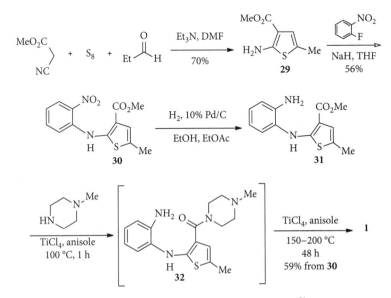

Scheme 1. The discovery synthesis of olanzapine (**1**)[24]

Alternatively, as shown in Scheme 2,[33, 34] substituting malononitrile with methyl cyanoacetate in the Gewald aminothiophene synthesis gave **29** with a carbometh-oxy group at the 3 position of the thiophene. Compound **29** was treated with 2-flu-oronitrobenzene to form **30** via an S_NAr coupling recation and hydrogenation of the nitro group provided **31**. The crude diamino ester was treated with *N*-methyl-piperazine in the presence of $TiCl_4$ at 100 °C for 1 h to give the intermediate amide **32**, which was heated under reflux for 48 h to effect ring closure to deliver **1**.

Scheme 2. An alternate synthesis of olanzapine (**1**)[31] ·

In 2013, a radiosynthesis of [^{11}C]-olanzapine (**1'**) was reported as a new potential PET 5-HT$_2$ and D$_2$ receptor radioligand.[35] As shown in Scheme 3, amidine **28** was treated with piperidine-carbamate **33** to give **34**. After removal of the *t*-butyl protecting group using TFA, the resulting desmethyl-olanzipine **21** was methylated with radiolabeled [^{11}C]-methyl triflate at 80 °C to deliver the desired PET reagent in 3 min.

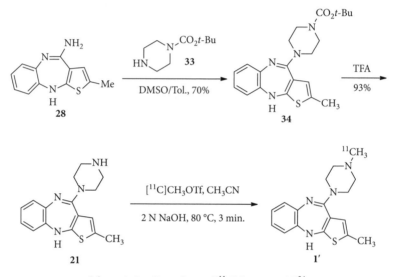

Scheme 3. A radiosynthesis of [^{11}C]olanzapine (**1'**)[34]

■ 4 CONCLUDING REMARKS

Schizophrenia is a devastating mental disorder without a cure to date. Despite the tremendous advances that we have made with atypical antipsychotics including Zyprexa (**1**), there is still a dire need for better treatments of schizophrenia that are short onset, highly efficacious, and devoid of the side effect of weight gain. Much is needed in this field. The patient is waiting.

■ 5 REFERENCES

1. Hirsch, S. R.; Weinberger, D. R. *Schizophrenia*, Blackwell Science: Malden, MA, 1995.

2. Brown, J. M.; Li, J. J.; Sinz, M. W. Antipsychotic Agents in *Burger's Medicinal Chemistry, Drug Discovery and Development*, 7th ed., Abraham, D. J.; Rotella, D. P., Eds.; Wiley: Hoboken, NJ, 2010, *Vol. 8*, pp. 161–218.

3. Li, J. J., *Laughing Gas, Viagra, and Lipitor, The Human Stories behind the Drugs We Use*, Oxford University Press: New York, 2006.

4. Healy, D. *The Creation of Psychopharmacology*, Harvard University Press: Cambridge, MA, 2004.

5. Ban, T. A. *Neuropsychiatr. Dis. Treat.* **2007**, *3*, 495–500.

6. Rees, L. *Br. Med. J.* **1960**, *2*, 522–525.

7. Granger, B.; Albu, S. *Ann. Clin. Psychiatry* **2005**, *17*, 137–140.

8. Arana, G. W. *J. Clin. Psychiatr.* **2000**, *61(Suppl. 8)*, 5–13.

9. Fitton, A.; Heel, R. *Drugs* **1990**, *40*, 722–747.

10. Casey, D. E.; Zorn, S. H. *J. Clin. Psychiatry*, **2001**, *62(Suppl. 7)*, 4–10.

11. Goodnick, P. J.; Jerry, J.; Parra, F. *Expert Opin. Pharmacother.* **2002**, *3*, 479–498.

12. Goodnick, P. J.; Rodriguez, L.; Santana, O. *Expert Opin. Pharmacother.* **2002**, *3*, 13814–13819.

13. Li, J. J.; Johnson, D. S.; Sliskovic, D. R.; Roth, B. D. *Contemporary Drug Synthesis*, Wiley: Hoboken, NJ, 2004, pp. 89–111.

14. Lowe, J. A., III CNS drugs, in *Drug Discovery: Practices, Processes, and Perspectives*, Li, J. J.; Corey, E. J., Eds.; Wileyr: Hoboken, NJ, 2012, pp. 245–286.

15. Meltzer, H. Y.; Matsubara, S.; Lee, J. *J. Pharmacol. Exp. Ther.* **1989**, *251*, 238–246.

16. Kuroki, T.; Nagao, N.; Nakahara, T. Neuropharmacology of second-generation antipsychotic drugs: a validity of the serotonin-dopamine hypothesis, in *Progress in Brain Research* 2008, *172 (Serotonin–Dopamine Interaction)*, Elsevier Science: Oxford 199–212.

17. Lund, B. C.; Perry, P. J. *Exp. Opin. Pharmacother.* **2000**, *1*, 305–323.

18. Kapur, S.; Seeman, P. *Am. J. Psychiatry* **2001**, *158*, 360–369.

19. Meltzer, H. Y.; Li, Z.; Kaneda, Y.; Ichikawa, J. *Prog. Neuropsychopharmacol. Biol. Psychiatry* **2003**, 27, 1159–1172.

20. Moore, N. A., Tupper, D. E., Hotten, T. M. *Drugs Fut.* **1994**, *19*, 114–117.

21. Kando, J. C.; Shepski, J. C.; Satterlee, W.; Patel, J. K.; Reams, S. G.; Green, A. I. *Ann. Pharmacother.* **1997**, *31*, 1325–1334.

22. Bhana, N.; Foster, R.; Olney, R.; Plosker, G. *Drugs* **2001**, *61*, 111–161.

23. Horacek, J.; Bubenikova-Valesova, V.; Kopecek, M.; Palenicek, T.; Dockery, C.; Mohr, P.; Hoschl, C. *CNS Drugs* **2006**, *20*, 389–409.

24. Chakrabarti, J. K.; Horsman, L.; Hotten, T. M.; Pullar, I. A.; Tupper, D. E.; Wright, F. C. *J. Med. Chem.* **1980**, *23*, 878–884.

25. Chakrabarti, J. K.; Hotten, T. M.; Morgan, S. E.; Pullar, I. A.; Rackham, D. M.; Risius, F. C.; Wedley, S.; Chaney, M. O.; Jones, N. D. *J. Med. Chem.* **1982**, *25*, 1133–1140.

26. Calligaro, D. O.; Fairhurst, J.; Hotten, T. M.; Moore, N. A.; Tupper, D. E. *Bioorg. Med. Chem. Lett.* **1997**, *7*, 25–30.

27. Zyprexa package insert. Eli Lilly & Co. (November 1998).

28. Kassahunk, K.; Mattiuz, Nyhart, E., Jr.; Obermeyer, B.; Gillespie, T.; Murphy, A.; Goodwin, R. M.; Tupper, D.; Callaghan, J. T.; Lemberger, L. *Drug Metab. Dispos.* **1997**, *25*, 81–93.

29. Ring, B. J.; Catlow, J.; Lindsay, T. J.; Gillespie, T.; Roskos, L. K.; Cerimele, B. J.; Swanson, S. P.; Hamman, M. A.; Wrighton, S. A. *J. Pharmacol. Exp. Ther.* **1996**, *276*, 658–666.

30. Tran, P. V.; Dellva, M. A.; Tollefson, G. D.; Beasley, C. M., Jr.; Potvin, J. H.; Kiesler, G. M. *J. Clin. Psychiatry* **1997**, *58*, 205–211.

31. Tohen, M.; Sanger, T. M.; Mcelroy, S. L. et al. *Psychiatry* **1999**, *156*, 702–709.

32. Chakrabarti, J. K.; Hicks, T. A.; Hotten, T. M. Tupper, D. E. *J. Chem. Soc. Perkin Trans. I* **1978**, 937–941.

33. Chakrabarti, J. K.; Hotten, T. M.; Tupper, D. E. US 5229382 (1993), EP 454436 (1991).

34. Chakrabarti, J. K.; Hotten, T. M.; Tupper, D. E. US 5627178 (1997).

35. Gao, M.; Shi, Z.; Wang, M.; Zheng, Q.-H. *Bioorg. Med. Chem. Lett.* **2013**, *23*, 1953–1956.

Drugs to Treat Infectious Diseases

9   Sofosbuvir (Sovaldi)

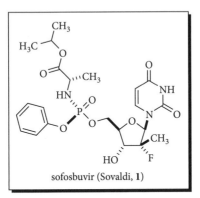

sofosbuvir (Sovaldi, **1**)

USAN:	*Sofosbuvir*
Brand Name:	*Sovaldi (Gilead)*
Molecular Weight:	*529.46*
FDA Approval:	*2013*
Drug Class:	*Phosphoramide Prodrug of Antiviral Nucelotide*
Indications:	*Hepatitis C Virus (HCV) Infection*
Mechanism of Action:	*HCV NS5B Polymerase Inhibitor*

▓ 1 HISTORY OF VIRUS AND ANTIVIRAL DRUGS

Viruses are humanity's invisible enemy. They wreak daily havoc by causing the flu, measles, rabies, hepatitis, smallpox, polio, and even human immunodeficiency virus (HIV). Although viruses have existed on the earth much longer than humans, it was not until in 1892 when the concept of virus took root when Chamberland experimented with viruses using the Pasteur–Chamberland filter. Solid evidence emerged when tobacco mosaic virus (TMV) crystal was isolated in 1935.

However, human ingenuity afforded successful measures to combat viruses long before 1892. For instance, Jenner successfully pioneered a vaccination for preventing smallpox in 1796, nearly one hundred years before Chamberland's exploits and before Pasteur developed the first vaccination for rabies in 1885. The scourge of polio has been nearly wiped out thanks to Salk's inactivated polio vaccine (IPV) available since 1954 and Sabin's oral poliovirus vaccine (OPV) popularized in 1960. The 1951 the Nobel Prize in Physiology or Medicine was awarded to Theiler for his contributions to yellow fever vaccines.

In terms of small molecule antiviral drugs, the nucleoside iododeoxyuridine (IDU, **2**), a simple analog of thymidine (**3**), was first synthesized and used as an antiviral drug in 1959 by Prusoff.[1] Unfortunately, due to its systemic cardiotoxicities, IDU is now only used topically to treat herpes simplex keratitis. A similar antiviral nucleoside, trifluorothymidine (TFT, Viroptic, 4), is less toxic than 2, and is also primarily used topically in eyes to kill the herpes simplex virus (HSV).[2]

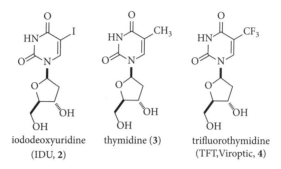

iododeoxyuridine (IDU, 2) thymidine (3) trifluorothymidine (TFT, Viroptic, 4)

Under the leadership of future Nobel laureate Elion, Burroughs Wellcome introduced the nucleoside analog acyclovir (Zovirax, 5) in 1978 for the treatment of HSV infection.[3] While not the first antiviral agent on the market, Zovirax (5) was the first small molecule drug to be widely used to control a viral infection. Introduction of valacyclovir (Valtrex, 6), a prodrug of Zovirax (5) with higher oral bioavailability, afforded the patient a more convenient regimen because it does not have to be taken as frequently as the parent drug Zovirax (5).[4] Coincidently the prodrug strategy employed here to improve oral bioavailability is a popular strategy in the antiviral drugs arena. The title antiviral drug sofosbuvir (Sovaldi, 1) is a prodrug as well.

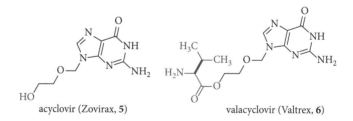

acyclovir (Zovirax, 5) valacyclovir (Valtrex, 6)

1.1 HIV Antiviral Drugs

Montagnier's discovery of the human immunodeficiency virus-1 (HIV-1) in 1983 earned him a Nobel Prize in 2008. Intensive efforts to fight the virus began as soon as acquired immunodeficiency syndrome (AIDS), caused by HIV, appeared at an alarming rate in the early 1980s. The National Institutes of Health (NIH) led a screening program by collecting compounds from major pharmaceutical companies. The first fruit of the pursuit was azidothymidine (zidovudine, AZT, 7), a sample submitted by Burroughs Wellcome. The nucleoside was initially prepared as an anticancer drug, but was shown to be an HIV reverse transcriptase inhibitor (RTI). In 1987, AZT (**7**) became the first antiretroviral agent approved for treating AIDS.[5] AZT (**7**) works by incorporation of AZT triphosphate into the growing DNA chain of DNA elongation and thus inhibits DNA synthesis.[6]

Similar to AZT (**7**), d4T (stavudine, **8**) was also first prepared as a potential anticancer agent and its HIV-1 inhibitory activity was revealed later. A newer drug, lamivudine (3TC, Epivir, **9**),[7] was discovered at Emory University and licensed to Glaxo. Antiviral drugs **7–9** all belong to the class of nucleoside reverse transcriptase inhibitors (NRTIs). They are also sometimes known as DNA chain terminators because of their MOA.

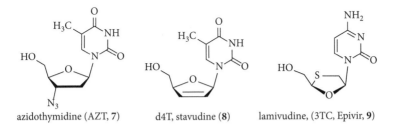

| azidothymidine (AZT, **7**) | d4T, stavudine (**8**) | lamivudine, (3TC, Epivir, **9**) |

Due to the mitochondrial toxicities often associated with NRTIs such as **7–9**,[8] rigorous efforts have been made to search for non-nucleoside reverse transcriptase inhibitors (NNRTIs).[9] The first three NNRTIs on the market at the end of 1990s were Boehringer–Ingelheim's neviripine (Viramune, **10**), Merck's efavirenz (Sustiva, **11**), and Upjohn/Pfizer's delavirdine mesylate (Rescriptor, **12**). Newer NNRTIs currently on the market as of 2014 include etravirine (Intelence) and rilpivirine (Edurant).[10]

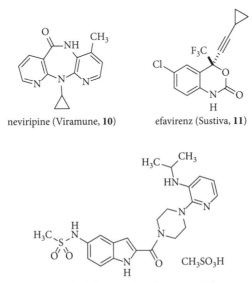

neviripine (Viramune, **10**)   efavirenz (Sustiva, **11**)

delavirdine mesylate (Rescriptor, **12**)

Perhaps the most visible achievement against AIDS was the emergence of HIV protease inhibitors (PIs) in the mid-1990s. A protease is an enzyme that breaks peptide bonds of the virus's proteins via hydrolysis. HIV protease is the enzyme that breaks the virus's polyprotein peptide bonds via hydrolysis, thus rendering the HIV virions noninfectious.

The first HIV protease inhibitor on the market, Roche's saquinavir (Invirase, **13**), was approved by the FDA in 1995 for the treatment of AIDS.[11] It was quickly followed by Abbott's ritonavir (Norvir)[12] and Merck's indinavir (Crixivan).[13] Nelfinavir (Viracept), amprenavir (Agenerase), fosamprenavir (Lexiva), lopinavir (Kelatra when combined with ritonavir), atazanavir (Reyataz), and tipranavir (Aptivus) have emerged since the 1990s. One of the latest HIV protease inhibitor is Merck's darunavir (Prezista, **14**). It was approved for the treatment of HIV/AIDS patients who are harboring drug-resistant HIV that does not respond to other therapies. The drug was discovered by Ghosh, who started the effort strictly as an educational project, at Purdue University.[14]

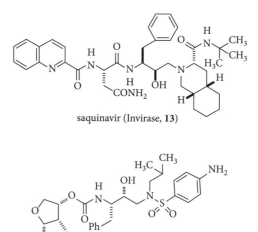

saquinavir (Invirase, **13**)

darunavir (Prezista, **14**)

In addition to HIV reverse transcriptase inhibitors (including both NRTIs and NNRTIs) and HIV protease inhibitors, several other novel MOA have afforded successful and alternative treatments in the clinics. Merck's raltegravir (Isentress, **15**) is the first FDA-approved inhibitor of HIV integrase.[15] Pfizer's maraviroc (Selzentry, **16**) is the first-in-class CCR5 antagonist for the treatment of HIV.[16]

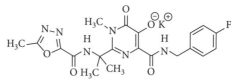

raltegravir (Isentress, **15**)

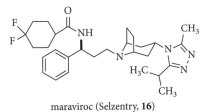

maraviroc (Selzentry, **16**)

1.2 Influenza Antiviral Drugs

Currently, there are four drugs available for the treatment or prophylaxis of influenza infections. The first two adamantanes include amantadine (Symmetrel, **17**) and rimantadine (Flumadine, **18**), which act as M_2 ion channel inhibitors and interfere with viral un-coating inside the cell.[17] They are effective only against influenza A and are associated with several toxic effects as well as drug resistance. They are now rarely used.

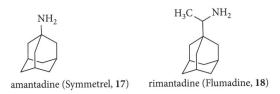

amantadine (Symmetrel, **17**)   rimantadine (Flumadine, **18**)

The influenza neuraminidase (also known as sialidase) is one of two major glycoproteins located on the influenza virus membrane envelope. The other glycoprotein is hemagglutinin. The combination of the variants of neuraminidase and hemagglutinin is used to name influenza strains, for example, N1H1 and N9H7. Two newer drugs to treat influenza are both neuraminidase inhibitors: oseltamivir (Tamiflu, **19**) and zanamivir (Relenza, **20**). They are kinder and gentler in comparison to adamantanes **17** and **18**. More important, they work better for both influenza A and B.

Oseltamivir (**19**), the first orally active neuraminidase inhibitor, is a prodrug. It was discovered by Gilead in 1995.[18] Gilead and Roche began co-developing it in 1995 and gained FDA approval in 1999. Zanamivir (**20**) is given via inhalation due to its poor oral bioavailability. It was discovered by Biota Holdings, a small Australian biotechnology concern.[19] In the United States, Biota established an alliance with GlaxoSmithKline for development and marketing of zanamivir (**20**), which was also approved by the FDA in 1999.

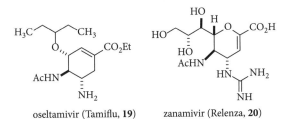

oseltamivir (Tamiflu, **19**)   zanamivir (Relenza, **20**)

1.3 Hepatitis Antiviral Drugs

Hepatitis B virus (HBV)[20] causes hepatitis in both humans and animals. Interferon and five nucleos(t)ides have been approved as treatments for chronic hepatitis B[21] in many parts of the world. Interferon, unfortunately, is effective only in a subset of HBV patients. Furthermore, it is often poorly tolerated, requires parenteral administration, and is expensive.[22] Lamivudine (3TC, Epivir, **9**) was the first oral antiviral drug for treating HBV. Tenofovir disoproxil fumarate (Viread, **21**) is an orally administered phosphate prodrug of tenofovir, an NRTI that shows potent in vitro activity against both HBV and HIV-1. Current treatments for HBV also include adefovir dipivoxil (Hepsera, **22**), Novartis's telbivudine (Tyzeka, **23**), BMS's entecavir (Baraclude, **24**), and the ever-versatile ribavirin (Rebetol, **25**), which has been used to treat hepatitis C virus (HCV) as well.

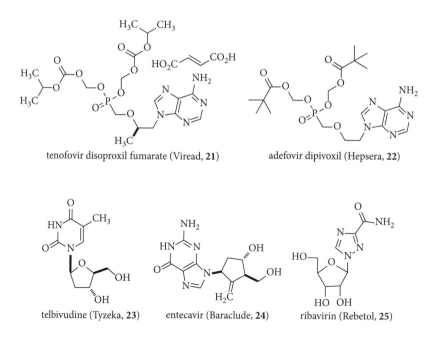

tenofovir disoproxil fumarate (Viread, **21**)   adefovir dipivoxil (Hepsera, **22**)

telbivudine (Tyzeka, **23**)   entecavir (Baraclude, **24**)   ribavirin (Rebetol, **25**)

Both **21** and **22** are prodrugs designed to boost the bioavailability of the parent drugs. For example, **21** is initially hydrolyzed by carboxyesterase to liberate one molecule of isopropanol and carboxylate **26**, as shown in Scheme 1.[23-25] Carboxylate **26** then spontaneously loses a molecule of CO_2 to provide another transient molecule **27**, which spontaneously loses a molecule of formaldehyde to provide phosphate **28**. Repeating the same sequence on the other side chain then delivers the active API as phosphoric acid **29**. Similar to AZT, **29** as a mono-phosphate is converted in vivo to **29**-ATP, which is the active species serving as a DNA chain terminator.

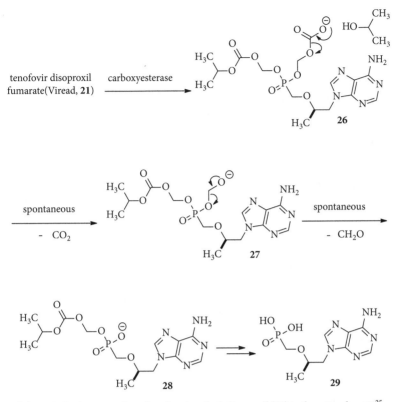

Scheme 1. *In vivo* conversion of prodrug tenofovir disoproxil (**21**) to the active drug **29**[25]

Hepatitis C, especially chronic hepatitis C, can severely damage the liver and cause liver carcinoma and eventually liver failure. More than 130 million people worldwide are infected with HCV.

Structurally, HCV has 10 proteins: three structural proteins and seven non-structural (NS) proteins. As shown in Fig. 9.1,[26] all the HCV enzymes including NS2/3 and NS3/4A proteases, NS3 helicase, NS5A, and NS5B RNA–dependent RNA polymerase (RdRp) are essential for HCV replication and have proven to be attractive targets for the development of anti-HCV therapy.

Older therapies for HCV infection include pegylated interferon-α (PEG-Intron) alone or in combination with ribavirin (Rebetol, **25**).[27] However, the antiviral activity of interferon is indirect, has to be given via IV, and possesses toxicities, often causing flu-like symptoms. Ribavirin (**25**) is a nonspecific agent with inhibitory activity toward some host proteins. Specifically targeted antiviral therapy for HCV would be more efficacious and have fewer side effects.[27] The resulting therapies include HCV NS2 and NS3/4 protease inhibitors, NS3 helicase inhibitors, NS4B and NS5A, and NS5B replication factor inhibitors, as well as HCV NS5B polymerase inhibitors. Sovaldi (**1**), the focus of this chapter, is a phosphoramide

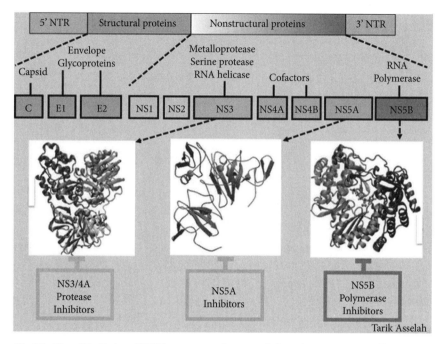

Fig. 9.1. Hepatitis C virus (HCV) genome and potential drug discovery targets.[26]
Reproduced with Permission

prodrug of an HCV NS5B polymerase inhibitor and belongs to the class of HCV NS5B polymerase inhibitors.

Excitingly, two oral anti-HCV drugs, both HCV NS3/4A serine protease inhibitors, were approved by the FDA in 2011: boceprevir (Victrelis, **30**),[28] by Schering–Plough/Merck, and telaprevir (Incivek, **31**),[29] by Vertex. These two innovative medicines were the first wave of safe, efficacious, and convenient treatment options for patients with HCV. Two years later, Janssen's simeprevir (Olysio, **32**), a second-generation protease inhibitor for the treatment of genotype 1 (G1) HCV infection, was approved by the FDA.[30] It is also an HCV NS3/4A serine protease inhibitor. Sovaldi (**1**) was also approved in 2013. Sovaldi (**1**) and the three HCV NS3/4A serine protease inhibitors **30–32** are also known as direct-acting antivirals (DAAs).

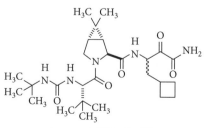

boceprevir (Victrelis, **30**)

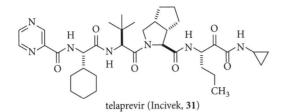

telaprevir (Incivek, **31**)

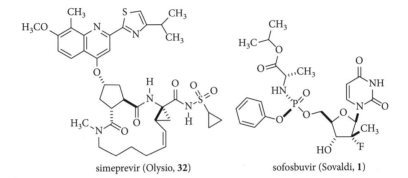

simeprevir (Olysio, **32**)   sofosbuvir (Sovaldi, **1**)

■ **2 PHARMACOLOGY**

2.1 Mechanism of Action

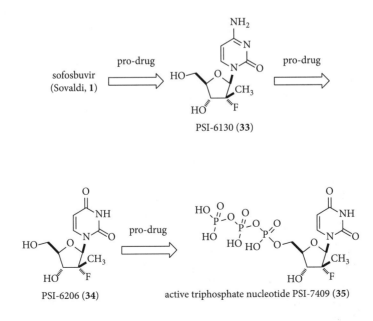

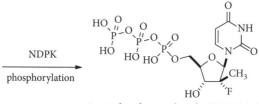

active triphosphate nucleotide PSI-7409 (**35**)

Scheme 2. Conversion of the phosphoramidate prodrug sofosbuvir
(**1**) to its active derivative PSI-7409 (**35**)[33]

Sovaldi (**1**) has a pan-genotypic antiviral effect although it might be less efficient in genotype 3 (G3). As a phosphoramide prodrug, it is not active in vitro. Instead, it undergoes extensive metabolisms in vivo under the influence of a battery of enzymes in the human body via a relatively complex activation pathway. The end product is a uridine triphosphate analog PSI-7409 (**35**). It is a potent HCV NS5B polymerase inhibitor in vitro. This active species is nucleotide analog (chain terminator) and is responsible for the drug's antiviral effects.

The inventor Pharmasset's initial significant contribution to the discovery of Sovaldi (**1**) was installation of the fluorine atom, affording a series of fluorine-containing nucleosides with unique *in vitro* and *in vivo* characteristics.[31] One of the company's early leads was 2'-α-fluoro-2'-β-methyl nucleoside PSI-6130 (**33**), which is a potent and selective inhibitor of HCV NS5B polymerase, which exhibited antiviral activity in cell culture systems with an EC_{90} of 4.6 μM in an HCV replicon assay and was efficacious in humans.[32] EC_{90} is the efficacious concentration that provokes a response that is 90% of the maximum; the smaller the EC_{90} value, the more potent the compound is.

Although PSI-6130 (**33**) was the first of this class to advance to clinical trials, it suffered from poor bioavailability. PSI-6206 (**34**), a metabolite of **33** by deamination of the cytosine, had a better PK profile. Despite the fact that PSI-6206 (**34**) is inactive in vitro (EC_{90} > 100 μM), its corresponding triphosphate form, PSI-7409 (**35**), is a potent inhibitor of HCV polymerase in *in vitro* assays.

The long and complicated metabolic pathway from Sovaldi (**1**) to its active form PSI-7409 (**35**) is shown in Scheme 2.[33-35] At first, Sovaldi (**1**) is converted to corresponding carboxylic acid **36** under the influence of human cathepsin A (CatA) and carboxylesterase 1 (CES1). Carboxylic acid **36** then undergoes a fast, non-enzymatic intramolecular nucleophilic attack to form a cyclic alaninyl phosphate intermediate **37**, which undergoes a hydrolysis of the cyclic phosphate to linear phosphate as carboxylic acid **38** with concomitant release of a molecule of phenol. Carboxylic acid **38** is further hydrolyzed by the histidine triad nucleotide-binding protein-1 (Hint1) enzyme to form monophosphate nucleotide **39**. It is phosphorylated to the diphosphate nucleotide **40** under the influence of uridine monophosphate-cytidine monophosphate (UMP-CMP) kinase. Finally, **40** is further phosphorylated to the active triphosphate nucleotide PSI-7409 (**35**) with the aid of nucleoside diphosphate kinase (NDPK).

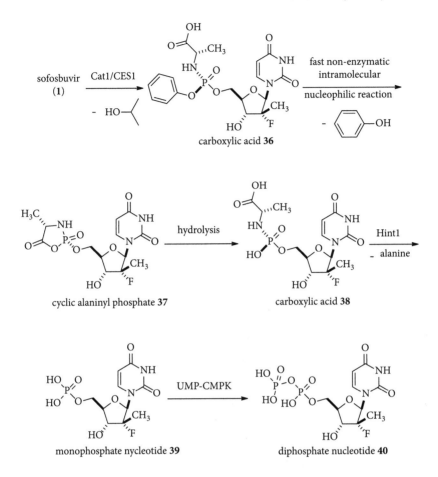

carboxylic acid **36**

cyclic alaninyl phosphate **37**

carboxylic acid **38**

monophosphate nycleotide **39**

diphosphate nucleotide **40**

2.2 Structure–Activity Relationship

Extensive SAR investigations were carried out with regard to the optimal substituents for the phosporamidate.[36] The final fine-tuning section of the SAR is summarized below (Table 9.1).

Pharmasset assessed their prodrugs' anti-HCV activity using the clone A replicon and a quantitative real-time PCR assay measured the EC_{90}. Each compound was also simultaneously evaluated for cytotoxicity by assessing the levels of cellular rRNA at 50 μM. Thus 0% would indicate the compound was devoid of cytotoxicity.

As shown in Table 9.1, when the ester moiety (R^1) on **41** was Me, Et, *i*-Pr, or Cy, compound **41** had submicromolar EC_{90} values. Although R^1 as *n*-Bu, *i*-Bu and *n*-pentane (not shown) afforded even more potent compounds; they also showed cytotoxicity and were thus not further pursued. Next, the α-substitution on alanine was altered.

As far as the R^2 on phosphoramidate **41** was concerned, 1-naphthyl ester (not shown) was the most potent compound, but its cytotoxicity (95.4% at 50 μM) was even

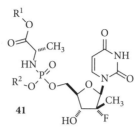

41

TABLE 9.1. *HCV Replicon Activity of Phosphoramidate Prodrugs: Simultaneous Carboxylate and Phenolic Ester Modification of the Phosphoramidate Moiety*[36]

compd	R¹	R²	EC_{90} clone A (μM)	inhibition of cellular rRNA replication at 50 μM (%)
41a	Me	Ph	1.62	0.0
41b	Me	4-F-Ph	0.69	16.8
41c	Me	4-Cl-Ph	0.58	62.8
41d	Me	4-Br-Ph	2.11	30.8
41e	Et	Ph	0.98	36.9
41f	Et	4-F-Ph	0.76	55.3
41g	Et	4-Cl-Ph	0.39	0.0
41h	Et	4-Br-Ph	0.36	80.5
41i	i-Pr	Ph	0.52	25.9
41j	i-Pr	4-F-Ph	0.77	0.0
41k	i-Pr	4-Cl-Ph	0.42	0.0
41l	i-Pr	4-Br-Ph	0.57	0.0
41m	Cy	Ph	0.25	61.1
41n	Cy	4-F-Ph	0.04	52.1
41o	Cy	4-Cl-Ph	0.054	66.9
41p	Cy	4-Br-Ph	0.039	91.5

higher than that of **41p** (91.5% at 50 μM). On the other hand, when R² was an *alkyl* group, the resulting compounds were not active. Therefore, the efforts of optimizing R² focused on simple phenyl or mono-halogenated phenyl substituents. Due the potential toxicities associated with poly-halogenated phenols, they were not considered.

On the basis of potency, safety, and structural considerations, seven compounds (**41a**, **41f**, **41i**, **41j**, **41k**, **41m**, and **41n**) from Table 9.2 were chosen for further evaluation. Among these compounds, **41a**, and **41i** produced the highest C_{max} (1985, 1934 ng/g) and AUC values (14206, 16796 ng•h/g), respectively.[36] Since **41i** had the highest plasma exposure in monkeys (>3-fold) than both **41a**, and **41n**, it was chosen to be advanced as their drug candidate. Compound **41i** is the mixture of diastereomers containing Sovaldi (**1**).

2.3 Bioavailability, Metabolism, and Toxicology

After separation of the two diastereomers of compound **41i** (see Section 3.1), Sovaldi (**1**) became available for further PK/PD studies. By design, the prodrug Sovaldi (**1**) is extensively metabolized by esterase activity, leading to relatively high exposure of the metabolites carboxylic acid **38** and PSI-6206 (**34**) in all tested species.[36]

Following oral administration of [^{14}C]-sofosbuvir (**1**) to rats,[32,33] the higher concentrations of radioactivity were observed in the organs of absorption and excretion and the lymphatic system. As shown in Scheme 3, carboxylic acid **38** is hydrolyzed to produce monophosphate nucleotide **39**, which has two pathways for metabolization. One is direct glucuronidation to give the corresponding glucuronide **42**. Meanwhile, portions of monophosphate nucleotide **39** is sulfated to make sulfate **43**. Both metabolites glucuronide **42** and sulfate **43** are significantly more polar than **39**, therefore, they are more readily eliminated or excreted through the system. Moreover, both rats and dogs had a urinary recovery accounting for 72% and 81%, respectively, of the administered radiolabeled material. PSI-6206 (**34**) was the predominant circulating metabolite, as well as the predominant metabolite in bile in rats and in urine and feces in both rats and dogs.[36]

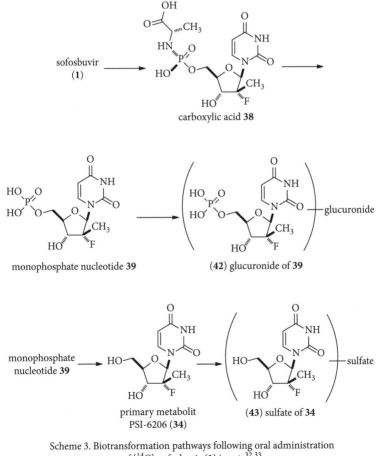

Scheme 3. Biotransformation pathways following oral administration of [^{14}C]-sofosbuvir (**1**) in rats[32,33]

When cynomolgus monkeys were given an oral dose of 50 mg/kg once daily for four days, the prodrug Sovaldi (**1**) had a C$_{max}$ 33 ng/mL and an AUC$_{(inf)}$ value of

170 ng•h/mL.[37] Bioavailability data in humans are scarce in literature because the drug is most often used in combination with ribavirin (**25**) and/or interferon.

Sovaldi is relatively safe. It is not metabolized by CYP450 enzymes (although it is metabolized by five other enzymes, as shown in Scheme 2), so it does not have the potential of DDIs with drugs that are metabolized by CYP450.[38] At the time of this writing (September 2014), Solvadi (**1**) has been on the market for nine months and has been proven to be reasonably safe. This is consistent with the preclinical/clinical studies where no major safety signal has been observed. Sovaldi (**1**) has no effect on QT_C so the potentials are low for the cardiac diseases associated with QT prolongation.

■ 3 SYNTHESIS

3.1 Discovery Route

Pharmasset published their discovery synthesis of the parent compound PSI-6206 (**34**) in 2005.[39]

PSI-6206's (**34**) precursor PSI-6130 (**33**) is only one carbon different from cytidine (**44**), the natural nucleoside. However, because this carbon is a fluorine-containing tertiary carbon, it makes the synthesis exponentially challenging. Pharmasset's medicinal chemists choose cytidine (**44**) as their starting material. As shown in Scheme 4, the aniline on cytidine (**44**) was benzoylated first, followed by treatment with tetra-isopropyldisiloxane-1,3-diyl-silyl chloride (TIDPSCl$_2$) and pyridine to give triple-protected **45**. The only exposed alcohol was oxidized using Swern-like conditions to afford a ketone, which was treated with methyllithium to produce tertiary alcohol **46**. Subsequently, the TIDPS protective group was removed by using the synergy between tetrabutylammonium fluoride (TBAF) and concentrated acetic acid. The exposed alcohols were reprotected as their benzoyl esters to give the globally protected intermediate **47**.

Treatment of tertiary alcohol **47** with diethylaminosulfur trifluoride (DAST) provided the fluorinated product **48** with inversion of configuration in 15–20% yield. This step was low-yielding because E_1 elimination of the alcohol on **47** gave the olefin as the major byproduct in addition to recovered starting material. Eventually, de-amination by refluxing **48** in 80% acetic acid was followed by removal of the remaining benzoyl protecting groups using methanolic ammonia to deliver PSI-6206 (**34**).

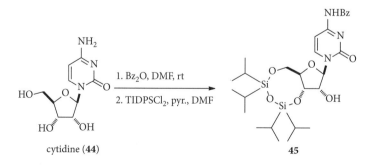

cytidine (**44**)   45

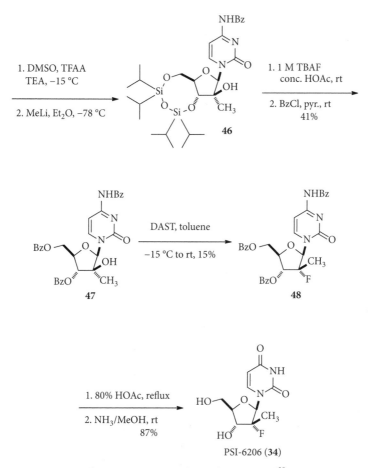

Scheme 4. Discovery synthesis of PSI-6206 (**34**)[39]

3.2 Intermediate Scale Route

The discovery route described in the previous section was sufficient to identify PSI-6206 (**34**) as the lead compound. While the synthesis was short (six steps), it required tedious chromatography steps and the DAST fluorination of alcohol **47** was very low yielding. In 2009, Pharmasset published their intermediate scale synthesis of PSI-6130 (**33**), a prodrug of PSI-6206 (**34**).[36,40]

In order to jump far, we sometimes have to back off a few steps. This is often the case for process chemistry: In order to come up with reproducible and easily operational large-scale synthesis, process chemists sometimes need to develop an optimal synthetic route that is actually longer than the discovery route. Here is an example.

As shown in Scheme 5, D-glyceraldehyde (**49**) was chosen as the starting material because it is inexpensive and readily available by oxidative cleavage of the diisopropylidene derivative of D-mannitol. The Wittig reaction of **49** with phosphorane **50** stereoselectively assembled olefin **51** with the *E*-olefin as the predominant geometrical isomer. Even without using the expensive Sharpless AD-mix-β, olefin **51** was stereoselectively dihydroxylated with $KMnO_4$ to give diol **52**. This is a classic case of substrate-directed asymmetric dihydroxylation.

Although cyclic sulfate **53** could be made in one step using sulfuryl chloride, it was found that a two-step procedure gave higher and more reproducible yields. Thus, diol **52** was converted to its corresponding cyclic sulfite followed by oxidation by sodium hypochlorite (bleach) with (2,2,6,6-tetramethylpiperidin-1-yl)oxy (TEMPO) as the catalyst.

Treatment of cyclic sulfate **53** with triethylammonium fluoride (TEAF) gave exclusively C-2 fluorination product **54**. Hydrolysis of a sulfate ester in the presence of an ester and acetonide is quite tricky because of the functional group compatibility issue. Here sulfate fluorohydrin **54** was treated with concentrated HCl *in the presence of 2,2-dimethoxypropane* (which reformed the acetonide) to provide fluorohydrin **55**. This step hydrolyzed the sulfate to the alcohol and kept the acetonide intact. Treatment of **55** with concentrated HCl in ethanol then gave rise to lactone diol **56** as a white solid in 67% yield from diol **52**.

Benzylation of lactone diol **56** with benzoyl chloride (BzCl) provided **57**. Reduction of lactone **57** was accomplished using the hindered reducing agent lithium tri-*tert*-butoxyaluminum hydride to afford lactol **58** as a 2:1 mixture of the β/α anomers. Lactol **58** was converted to its corresponding acetate **59**, which was better for the next coupling reaction with silylated N^4-benzoylcytosine **60**. The best conditions for the subsequent coupling reaction between acetate **59** and **60** used the Lewis acid, stannic chloride, as a mediator, and chlorobenzene as the solvent at 65 °C to give adduct **61**. Compound **61** was then treated with methanolic ammonia to provide the parent drug PSI-6130 (**33**) in 78% yield.

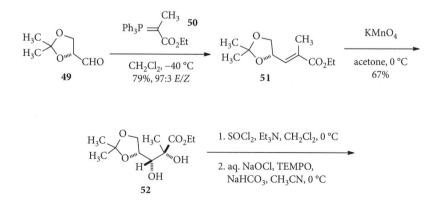

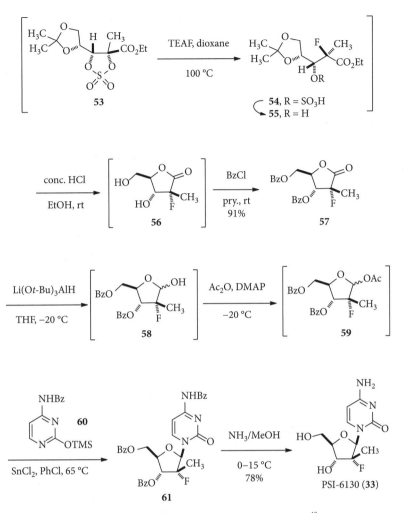

Scheme 5. Intermediate scale synthesis of PSI-6130 (33)[40]

In summary, Pharmasset's intermediate-scale synthesis produced PSI-6130 (33) in an overall yield of 6.4% from the Wittig reagent 50. No chromatography was used during the process because three intermediates are solids: diol 56, protected lactone 57, and the protected tribenzoylated product 61.

Pharmasset's synthesis of Sovaldi (1) used PSI-6206 (34) as the intermediate.[36] As shown in Scheme 6, the isopropyl ester of alanine (62) was coupled with phenyl phosphorodichloridate to give phosphoryl chloride 63 with the aid of N-methyl-imidazole (NMI). The installation of the prodrug moiety 63 onto the parent drug PSI-6206 (34) was also aided by NMI to afford adduct 41i as a 1:1 mixture of diastereomers at the phosphorus center of the phosphoramidate moiety. Preparatory-HPLC separation gave rise to two doastereomers 1 and 1'. The single crystal X-ray structure of **1** was obtained to establish the absolute configuration of the phosphorus center as S_p. By deference, the configuration of **1'** is R_p. In the clone A replicon assay, compounds **1'** and **1** produced anti-HCV activity with EC_{90} values of 7.5 and 0.42 μM, respectively. Therefore, the S_p diastereomer **1** is 17-fold more potent than the corresponding R_p diastereomer **1'**. This was the first example where stereochemistry at phosphorus could be correlated unequivocally to nucleotide phosphoramidate activity.

The S_p diastereomer **1** was assigned a code name PSI-7977, and was later granted an USAN (United States Adopted Name) of sofosbuvir. It became GS-7977 after Gilead purchased Pharmasset. Sofosbuvir gained regulatory approval in 2013 and Gilead sold it under the trade name Sovaldi.

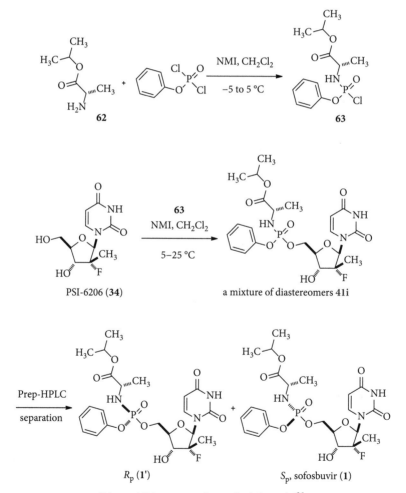

Scheme 6. Discovery synthesis of sofosbuvir (**1**)[36]

3.3 Process Route

Further process development of the route described in Section 3.2 led to the multikilogram clinical material production with the most notable improvement at the glycosylation step (59%) and an overall yield over 20%.[41]

As shown in Scheme 7, the asymmetric dihydroxylation of olefin **51** was found to be best carried out with *sodium* permanganate instead of *potassium* permanganate to prepare diol **52**. Sodium bisulfite was then used to quench the excess oxidant after the reaction. Cyclic sulfite **64** was prepared similar to the intermediate scale route (see Section 3.2) and was further oxidized to the corresponding sulfate **53** using sodium hypochlorite (bleach). Treating **53** with triethylamine–trihydrofluoride salt in the presence of triethylamine at 85 °C gave rise to sulfate fluorohydrin **65**. It was promptly hydrolyzed to afford the corresponding triol, which instantaneously cyclized to γ-lactone diol **56**. Protection of the diol was accomplished using benzoyl chloride (BzCl) to give **57**. Since **57** is a solid, it offered a good juncture for recrystallization.

Red-Al [sodium bis(2-methoxyethoxy)aluminum hydride] was employed to selectively reduce lactone **57** to lactol **58**, which was converted to chloride **61** as the key coupling partner. The coupling between chloride **66** and *O*-trimethyl silyl-N^4-benzoylcytosin (**60**) was promoted by stannic chloride to produce adduct **61**. Finally, global deprotection of **61** using catalytic amount of methanolic sodium methoxide in methanol then delivered desired PSI-6130 (**33**).

Currently in the US, a full course of treatment of Sovaldi (**1**) costs $84,000, which translates to approximately $1,000 per pill. There are numerous factors influencing pricing. From the chemistry perspective, the cost of good (CoG) and the long and tedious manufacturing process certainly is one of the factors that render the drug so expensive.

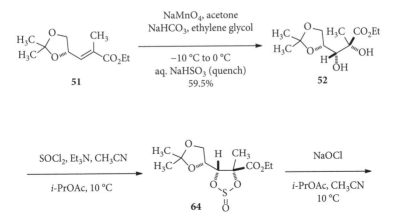

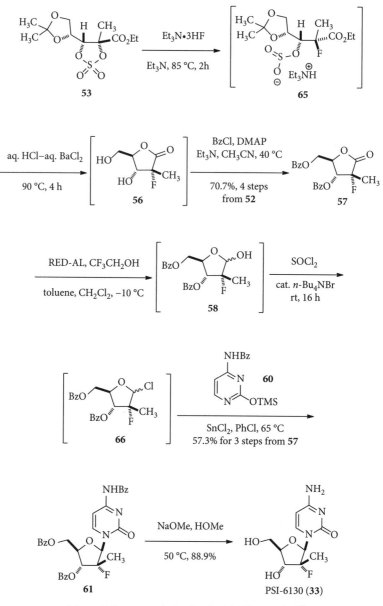

Scheme 7. Process synthesis of nucleotide PSI-6130 (**33**)[41]

■ **4 CONCLUDING REMARKS**

Newer and better medicines for the treatment of HCV infection is a new frontier for the pharmaceutical industry, with each having the potential to be a blockbuster drug. Many resources have been invested in this field and the fruits of those endeavors are emerging as one of the few bright aspects for the battered drug industry. Sovaldi (**1**) was projected to have sales of $5 billion in the first quarter after its introduction in 2014. Certainly, development of anti-HCV drugs can help slow the decline—perhaps even heralding the renaissance of drug discovery.

■ 5 REFERENCES

1. Prusoff, W. H. *Biochim. Biophys. Acta* **1959**, *32*, 295–296.

2. O'Brien, W.; Taylor, J. *Invest. Ophthalmol. Vis. Sci.* **1991**, *32*, 2455–2461.

3. Elion, G. B.; Furman, P. A.; Fyfe, J. A.; De Miranda, P.; Beauchamp, L.; Schaeffer, H. J. *PNAS* **1977**, *74*, 5716–5720.

4. Ormrod, D.; Goa, K. *Drugs* **2000**, 59, 1317–1340.

5. Broder, S. *Antiviral Res.* **2010**, *85*, 1–18.

6. Furman, P. A.; Fyfe, J. A.; St. Clair, M. H. et al. *PNAS* **1986**, *83*, 8333–8337.

7. Borman, S. *Chem. Eng. News* **2007**, *85*, 42–47.

8. Van Huyen, J.-P. D.; Landau, A.; Piketty, C.; Bélair, M.-F.; Batisse, D.; Gonzalez-Canali, G.; Weiss, W.; Jian, R.; Michel D. Kazatchkine, M. D.; Bruneval, P. *Am. J. Clin. Pathol.* **2003**, 119, 546–555.

9. De Clercq, E. *Adv. Pharm.* **2013**, *67 (Antiviral Agents)*, 317–358.

10. Song, Y.-n.; Fang, Z.; Zhan, P.; Liu, X. *Curr. Med. Chem.* **2014**, *21*, 329–355.

11. Duncan, I. B.; Redshaw, S. *Infect. Disease Ther.* **2002**, *25*, 27–47.

12. Kempf, D. J. *Infect. Disease Ther.* **2002**, *25*, 49–64.

13. Dorsey, B. D.; Vacca, J. P. *Infect. Disease Ther.* **2002**, *25*, 65–83.

14. Ghosh, A. K.; Martyr, C. D. in *Modern Drug Synthesis,* Li, J. J.; Johnson, D. S., Eds., Wiley: Hoboken, NJ, 2010, pp. 29–144.

15. Hunt, J. A., in *Modern Drug Synthesis,* Li, J. J.; Johnson, D. S., Eds., Wiley: Hoboken, NJ, 2010, pp. 315.

16. Price, D., in *Modern Drug Synthesis,* Li, J. J.; Johnson, D. S., Eds., Wiley: Hoboken, NJ, 2010, pp. 1728.

17. Kolocouris, N.; Kolocouris, A.; Foscolos, G. B.; Fytas, G.; Padalko, E.; Neyts, J.; De Clercq, E. *Biomed. Health Res.* **2002**, *55*, 103–115.

18. Lew, W.; Chen, X.; Kim, C. U. *Curr. Med. Chem.* **2000**, *7*, 663–672.

19. Smith, P. W.; Sollis, S. L.; Howes, P. D.; Cherry, P. C.; Starkey, I. D.; Cobley, K. N.; Weston, H.; Scicinski, J.; Merritt, A.; Whittington, A. et al. *J. Med. Chem.* **1998**, *41*, 787–797.

20. Meanwell, N. A.; D'Andrea, S. V.; Cianci, C. W.; Dicker, I. B.; Yeung, K.-S.; Belema, M.; Krystal, M. *Antiviral Drugs* In *Drug Discovery,* Li, J. J.; Corey, E. J., Eds.; Wiley: Hoboken, NJ, 2013, pp. 439–515.

21. Lok, A. S.-F. *Hepatol.* **2013**, *58*, 483–485.

22. Wan, M. B.; Weng, X. H. *J. Digest. Disease* **2013**, *14*, 626–637.

23. Shaw, J.-P.; Sueoka, C. M.; Oliyai, R.; Lee, W. A.; Arimilli, M. N.; Kim, C. U.; Cundy, K. C. *Pharm. Res.* **1997**, *14*, 1824–1829.

24. Li, F.; Maag, H.; Alfredson T. *J. Pharm. Sci.* **2008**, *97*, 1109–1034.

25. Filho, R. P.; Polli, M.; Filho, S. B.; Garcia, M.; Ferreira, E. I. *Braz. J. Pharm. Sci.* **2010**, *46*, 527–536.

26. Asselah, T.; Marcellin, P. *Liver Int.* **2013**, *33*, 93–104.

27. Meanwell, N. A.; Kadow, J. F.; Scola, P. M. *Ann. Rep. Med. Chem.* **2009**, *44*, 397–440.

28. Venkatraman, S. *Trends Pharmacol. Sci.* **2012**, *33*, 289–294.

29. Matthews, S. J.; Lancaster, J. W. *Clin. Therapeut.* **2012**, *34*, 1857–1882.

30. You, D. M.; Pockros, P. J. *Expert Opin. Pharmacother.* **2013**, *14*, 2581–2589.

31. Sofia, M. J.; Chang, W.; Furman, P. A.; Mosley, R. T.; Ross, B. S. *J. Med. Chem.* **2012**, *55*, 2481–2531.

32. Rodriguez-Torres, M. *Exp. Rev. Anti-Infect. Ther.* **2013**, *1*, 1269–1279.

33. Murakami, E.; Tolstykh, T.; Bao, H. et al. *J. Biol. Chem.* **2010**, *285*, 34337–34347.

34. Sofia, M. J. *Antiviral Chem. Chemother.* **2011**, *22*, 23–49.

35. Lam, A. M.; Murakami, E.; Espiritu, C. et al. *Antimicrob. Agents Chemother.* **2010**, *54*, 3187–3196.

36. Sofia, M. J.; Bao, D.; Chang, W. et al. *J. Med. Chem.* **2010**, *53*, 7202–7218.

37. *Sofosbuvir Investigator's Brochure, Edition 5*, Section 3.2, 33–45. Gilead Sciences

38. Asselah, T. *Exp. Opin. Pharmacother.* **2014**, *15*, 121–130.

39. Clark, J. L.; Hollecker, L.; Mason, J. C. et al. *J. Med. Chem.* **2005**, *48*, 5504–5508.

40. Wang, P.; Chin, B.-K.; Rachakonda, S.; Du, J.; Khan, N.; Shi, J.; Stec, W.; Cleary, D.; Ross, B. S.; Sofia, M. J. *J. Org. Chem.* **2009**, *74*, 6819–6824.

41. Axt, S.; Chun, B.-K.; Jin, Q.; Rachakonda, S.; Ross, B.; Sarma, K.; Vitale, J.; Zhu, J. EP20070839369 (2007). Intl. Pat Appl. WO 2008/045419 (2008).

Ulcer Drugs

10   Esomeprazole (Nexium)

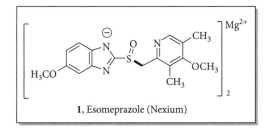

1, Esomeprazole (Nexium)

USAN:	*Esomeprazole*
Brand Name:	*Nexium (AstraZeneca)*
Molecular Weight:	*713.13*
FDA Approval:	*2001*
Drug Class:	*Anti-Ulcer*
Indications:	*Gastroesophageal Reflux Disease (GERD)*
Mechanism of Action:	*Proton Pump Inhibitor (H^+/K^+-ATPase Inhibitor)*

■ 1 HISTORY OF ULCER AND ULCER DRUGS

Gastric acid, hydrochloric acid (HCl), is essential to our digestion. It helps break down proteins, fats, and starches in our food into nutrients such as amino acids and carbohydrates that our body can absorb. Alas, there can be too much of a good thing. Too much secretion of gastric acid for too long can cause heartburn or acid reflux, also known as gastroesophageal reflux disease (GERD). In addition, having too much gastric acid for too long will damage the mucosa of the stomach and may cause ulcer and even stomach cancers!

While the exact pathogenesis of ulcers is not known, theories abound. It is still a popular belief that ulcer is caused by stress. Thirty years ago, the discovery of *Helicobacter pylori* demonstrated that the bacterium contributes to gastritis and peptic ulcers.[1]

Regardless of the root of stomach ulcers, they are closely associated with excessive secretion of gastric acid, so that was what early ulcer drugs intended to treat. Dozens of antacids are on the market to neutralize excess HCl: For instance, Mylanta and Maalox contain $Al(OH)_3$ and $Mg(OH)_2$. Tums contains $CaCO_3$. Alka-Seltzer contains $NaHCO_3$ (baking soda).

However, antacids only treat the symptoms of excessive acid secretion, and are therefore only effective as a short-term treatment. A better therapy would treat the causation of excessive acid secretion. Histamine-2 receptor antagonists work by blocking the receptors that are responsible for excessive acid secretion: the histamine-2 receptors. As a consequence, they are more efficacious and have fewer adverse effects in comparison to conventional antacids.

1.1 Histamine-2 Receptor Antagonists

The fact that histamine stimulates gastric acid secretion in the stomach was first observed by Popielski in the 1920s.

Popielski studied under Pavlov, who won the Nobel Prize (for Physiology or Medicine) in 1904 for his studies in digestive system, but who is now better known for his classical dog-conditioning experiments. As an independent researcher at the University of Kraków, Popielski discovered that histamine was a stimulant of gastric glands, and acted directly without the involvement of vagal nerves.[2] After injecting histamine subcutaneously into gastric fistulas in dogs, Popielski observed copious gastric acid secretion and extremely high acidity in the dogs' stomachs.[3] The experiment solidly established the association between histamine and gastric acid secretion.

Interestingly enough, antihistamines used to treat allergies did not have significant impact on gastric acid secretion. This observation led Black at SmithKline & French (SK&F) to speculate in 1964 that there were two types of histamine receptors, and that selective histamine H_2 receptor antagonists would be effective in decreasing gastric acid secretion and treating peptic ulcer.[4] The fruit of SK&F's endeavor was cimetidine (Tagamet, 2), which revolutionized the treatment of peptic ulcers. However, cimetidine (2), the prototype for H_2 receptor antagonists, had a trio of shortcomings: short half-life, DDI, and occasionally causing gynecomastia in some male patients due to its antiandrogenic activities. Ranitidine (Zantac, 3), famotidine (Pepcid, 4), and nizatidine (Axid, 5) are more potent and more selective and also safer than cimetidine (2). They (3–5) are devoid of the trio of the drawbacks associated with cimetidine (2).[5-7]

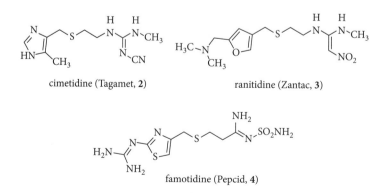

cimetidine (Tagamet, **2**) ranitidine (Zantac, **3**)

famotidine (Pepcid, **4**)

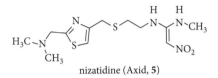

nizatidine (Axid, **5**)

The H$_2$ receptor antagonist approach produced many blockbuster drugs that revolutionized the pharmaceutical industry. Cimetidine (Tagamet, **2**), in fact, was the first blockbuster drug, with annual sales over $1 billion.

1.2 Proton Pump Inhibitors

While H$_2$ receptor antagonist approach were succeeding, other MOAs in treating ulcer were being pursued by many pharmaceutical companies. Hässle AB Sweden (now AstraZeneca) began their Gastrin Project in 1967. At the time, the *rational drug design* approach in drug discovery was not yet popular. Hässle tackled their Gastrin Project the old fashioned way: using animal models. Basically, they prepared compounds and tested them in fistula in dogs to see if the compound lowered the acidity of the dog's stomach.[8]

Hässle first derived their inspirations from Servier's CMN 131 (**6**), a thioamide and SK&F's cimetidine (**2**) to arrive at H 77/67 (**7**) with an imidazoline moiety.[9,10] Moving away from thioamide was understandable because of thioamide's propensity to cause hepatotoxicity.[11] Further development led to H 124/26 (**8**), which was unfortunately covered by a Hungarian patent. Fortuitously, its oxidative metabolite H 83/69 (timoprazole, **9**) was even more active than sulfide **8**. Unfortunately, timoprazole (**9**) was associated with thymus and thyroid toxicities. Hässle prepared picoprazole (**10**) in 1976.

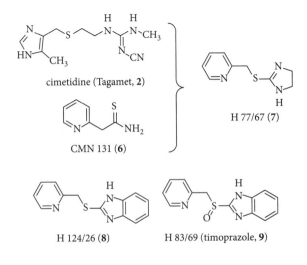

cimetidine (Tagamet, **2**)

CMN 131 (**6**)

H 77/67 (**7**)

H 124/26 (**8**)

H 83/69 (timoprazole, **9**)

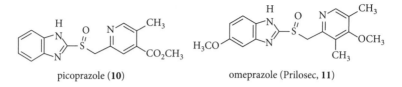

picoprazole (**10**)   omeprazole (Prilosec, **11**)

Picoprazole (**10**) was later found to cause necrotizing vasculitis in the small in-testine in some dogs when given too much for too long.[12] Efforts were made to find safer analogs of picoprazole (**10**). Since 3,5-dimethyl-4-methoxy-pyridine was known to increase the basicity of a pyridine ring, Hässle prepares it without sys-tematically explore the SAR. Omeprazole (**11**) tested as the most powerful inhib-itor of stimulated gastric acid secretion in experimental animals at the time. The drug had no sign of serious toxicity in animal models.

Omeprazole (Prilosec, **11**) was approved by the FDA in 1990 and was the world's best-selling drug from 1996 to 2000, when it was unseated by atorvastatin calcium (Lipitor; see chapter 1).

Lansoprazole (Prevacid, **12**) is another proton pump inhibitor (PPI) sold by TAP Pharmaceuticals, a joint venture of Abbott Laboratories and Takeda. Two other PPIs are pantoprazole (Protonix, **13**) and rabeprazole (Aciphex, **14**).[13]

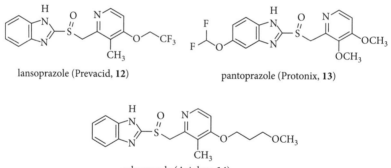

lansoprazole (Prevacid, **12**)   pantoprazole (Protonix, **13**)

rabeprazole (Aciphex, **14**)

In 1987, a group at Hässle embarked on a focused program to find a backup for Prilosec (**11**) with better bioavailability. Among all the compounds, only one was better than Prilosec: the S-(–)-diastereomer of omeprazole, esomeprazole (Nexium, **1**). When tested in rats, Nexium was 4–5 times more bioavailable than the R-diaste-reomer (**1′**).[14] Another lucky break for Hässle was that they tested Nexium (**1**) di-rectly in humans and saw similar effects to what they observed with rats. Later, when the two isomers were tested on dogs, no significant difference of efficacy was detected for the two isomers. In this case, rat was a better animal model than dog: Had they used dogs for their initial *in vivo* tests, they probably would never have found Nexium (**1**).[15]

Just as Prilosec's patent was about to expire, AstraZeneca launched Nexium (**1**) in early 2001. The timing generated some controversy with regard to whether

Prilosec (**11**) and Nexium (**1**) become the same molecule in the human body after metabolism. We will address the issue in the remainder of the chapter.

Nexium was the best-selling drug of the year in 2012 with annual sales of $6 billion. However, it lost patent protection in 2014.

■ 2 PHARMACOLOGY

2.1 Mechanism of Action

The MOA of Nexium (**1**) is through inhibition of an enzyme called gastric H+/K+-ATPase, also known as proton pump.

In the late 1970s, Sachs's group showed that H+/K+-ATPase was the proton pump of the stomach.[16] They also described immunologic detection of the pump in different organs using a polycolonal antibody against the ATPase. The enzyme reacted strongly with the stomach and weakly with the thyroid. In 1978, collaborating with Hässle, Sachs demonstrated that timoprazole (**8**) and picoprazole (**9**) were prodrugs but were converted to the active form after accumulation in the acidic secretory canaliculus of the parietal cells. "Thus arose an entirely new domain of peptic ulcer therapy," claimed Modlin, a professor at Yale Medical School. [17]

Similar to timoprazole (**8**) and picoprazole (**9**), omeprazole (**10**) itself is not active in inhibiting the ATPase in vitro. Rather, it is also a prodrug and becomes activated in vivo via the "omeprazole cycle" as shown in Scheme 1.[18,19] Sequentially, protonation of **10** takes place slowly when it encounters the acidic medium in the stomach. The protonated benzimidazole intermediate **14** then undergoes an intramolecular nucleophilic cyclization in a 5-*exo-dig* fashion where the pyridine moiety serves as the nucleophile to furnish benzimidazoline **15**. A reversible ring opening of **15** then delivers sulfenic acid **16**, which serves as an electrophile in a 6-*exo-trig* ring-closure to afford the reactive sulfenamide intermediate **17** after dehydration. The sulfenamide **17** is a very good electrophile, and is readily attacked by the cysteine residue of the enzyme H+/K+-ATPase. Therefore, Prilosec (**11**) is a pro-drug and sulfenamide **17** is the actual inhibitory species.

Nexium (**1**) is the (*S*)-enantiomer of racemic Prilosec (**11**), which is a mixture of two enantiomers. The former has better pharmacokinetics and pharmacodynamics than the latter and therefore possesses higher efficacy in controlling acid secretion and has a better therapeutic profile (see below).

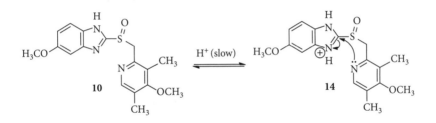

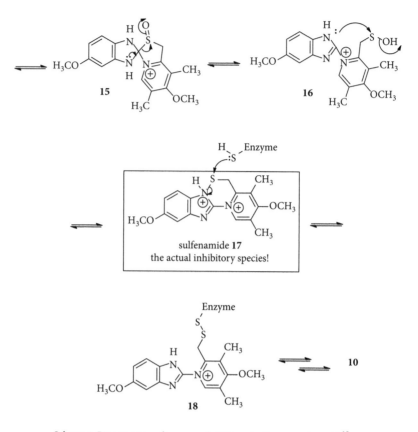

Scheme 1. Bioactivation of omeprazole (**10**) — the "omeprazole cycle"[18]

2.2 Structure–Activity Relationship

The SAR of Prilosec (**11**) was extensively investigated.[14] An abridged SAR table is shown in Table 10.1. The inhibitory effect of some Prilosec analogs on a partially purified H⁺/K⁺-ATPase is represented as pIC_{50}, which is the negative logarithm of its corresponding IC_{50} values. Meanwhile, pSA (SA stands for the quantity of sulfonamide, e.g., sulfenamide **17** in Fig. 10.1) is the negative logarithm of quantity (in mol/L of incubation mixture) of sulfenamide needed for 50% inhibition.[20]

From the earlier SAR, a generic structure of **19** possessing a substituted pyridine and a substituted benzimidazole was found to be the required core structure to have the antisecretory effect. When the Hässle team attempted to replace either pyridine or benzimidazole with other heterocycles, they observed no significant boost of the gastric acid inhibitory effect. Only a few close analogs of the benzimidazole, such as imidazole and aza-benzimidazole, showed weak inhibitory ability. This is readily explained using the "omeprazole cycle" because both pyridine and benzimidazole work in tandem to form the reactive sulfenamide intermediate such as **17**.

TABLE 10.1. *Inhibitory effect of some omeprazole analogs on a partially purified H^+/K^+-ATPase*[20]

Entry	Compound	R^1	R^2	Drug decomposed to SA in 30 min (%)	pIC_{50}	pSA
1	19a	3,5-$(CH_3)_2$,4-CH_3O	H	9.6	6.2	7.2
2	10	3,5-$(CH_3)_2$,4-CH_3O	5-CH_3O	7.8	5.7	6.8
3	19b	3,5-$(CH_3)_2$,4-CH_3O	5-Cl	13.2	6.2	7.1
4	19c	3,5-$(CH_3)_2$,4-CH_3O	5-$(CH_3)_2CH$	11.4	6.1	7.0
5	19d	3,5-$(CH_3)_2$,4-CH_3O	5-CH_3SO	61.2	6.6	6.8
6	19e	3,5-$(CH_3)_2$,4-CH_3O	5-CH_3CONH	6.6	5.7	6.9
7	19f	3,5-$(CH_3)_2$,4-CH_3O	5-NO_2	100	6.7	6.7
8	19g	H	5-CH_3O	1.0	5.1	7.1
9	19h	4-CH_3	5-CH_3O	2.4	5.2	6.8
10	19i	5-C_2H_5	5-CH_3O	1.3	5.0	6.9
11	19j	4,5-$(CH_3)_2$	5-CH_3O	5.1	5.1	7.5
12	19k	3,4,5-$(CH_3)_3$	5-CH_3O	16.4	6.5	7.3
13	19l	3,5-$(CH_3)_2$,4-C_2H_5O	5-CH_3O	6.9	5.7	6.9

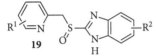

The sulfur atom was ideal to be a sulfoxide. Both sulfide and sulfone were inactive in vitro. One-carbon linkers ($-CH_2S-$, $-CH_2SO-$, and $-CH(CH_3)SO-$) all showed antisecretory activity in vivo. The fact that the sulfide is active in vivo is apparently due to its oxidation to the sulfoxide by CYP450. Elongating the linker between the sulfoxide and the pyridine did not offer any advantages, so one carbon linker was kept constant.

In entries 1–7, the pyridine rings with 3,5-$(CH_3)_2$, 4-CH_3O substituents seem to be optimal. Because 3,5-dimethyl-4-methoxy-pyridine was known to increase the basicity of a pyridine ring, Hässle prepared it without systematically exploring the SAR. The result was that the pK_a values of the pyridine ring was increased and the compounds containing the 3,5-dimethyl-4-methoxy-substituents were found to be most potent. This could also be explained by the omeprazole cycle. Since 3,5-dimethyl-4-methoxy-pyridine is the most basic, **14** *donates* electron pairs with the greatest ease, thus promoting the catalytic cycle. As luck would have it, later systemic SAR studies demonstrated that 3,5-dimethyl-4-methoxy-pyridine had higher *in vivo* potency than the corresponding 3-methyl-4-methoxy-pyridine and 5-methyl-4-methoxy-pyridine analogs.[14]

Substituents on the benzimidazole have a less profound impact on the potency of drugs. In entry 7, nitro compound **19f** completely (100%) converted to the active sulfenamide (SA, similar to **17**) within 30 min after dosing. It is possible that the nitro group is strongly electron-withdrawing, rendering the benzimidazole more prone to *accept* an electron pair from the pyridine ring, thus accelerating the catalytic cycle. Not surprisingly, another electron-withdrawing group methylsulfoxide showed similar acceleration of SA formation, albeit to a lesser extent. However, **19f** was not chosen as a development candidate. It can be speculated that nitro-aromatics have been historically associated with liver toxicities so that a conscious decision was probably made to avoid it. In the end, 5-methoxy-substitution of benzimidazole (entry 2) was chosen not only because **10** is potent, but also based on other pharmaceutics considerations, such as stability, crystallinity, and the ease with which to handle the active pharmaceutical ingredient (API).

2.3 Bioavailability, Metabolism and Toxicology

Not surprisingly, the bioavailabilities of both Prilosec (**11**) and Nexium (**1**) are complicated by the fact that they are prodrugs and the original APIs are completely metabolized in vivo once they come in contact with gastric acid.[21-26] This argues for the merit of using animal models rather than rational drug design, which may not find Prilosec (**11**) in the first place.

First-pass metabolism, sometimes also known as first-pass elimination, takes place largely in the liver where CYP450 enzymes oxidize the drug and make it more polar, and thus easier to eliminate. In clinical trials with young healthy volunteers, only 54% of a given dose of Prilosec (**11**) remained after dosing due to extensive first-pass metabolism.[21] This means that within a couple of hours dosing, nearly half of the API has been absorbed and eliminated.[22]

Three major metabolism pathways for Prilosec (**11**) are shown in Fig. 10.1.[23-25] All three are oxidative processes. On the left of the figure, under the influence of S-mephenytoin hydroxylase (S-MPH) and CYP3A, the 5-methyl group on the

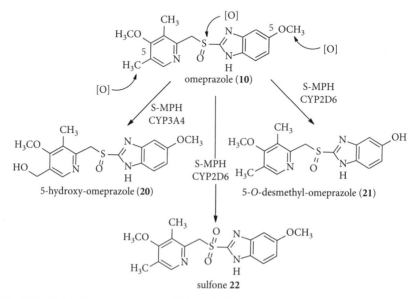

Fig. 10.1. Metabolism of omeprazole (**10**) in vivo[21]

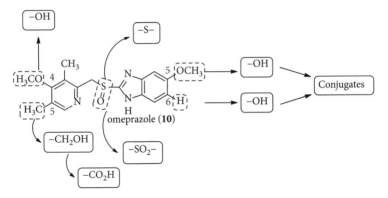

Fig. 10.2. Summary of Metabolism of Omeprazole (10)[21]

pyridine ring of omeprazole (**10**) is oxidized to the corresponding pyridylmethyl alcohol (**20**), which could be potentially further oxidized to the corresponding acid (see Fig. 10.2). Meanwhile, O-demethylation of the 4-methoxyl group on the pyridine ring provides a metabolite as 4-hydroxypyridine, which is unstable in the physiological environment.

One of the major first-pass metabolism of Prilosec (**11**) is hydroxylation by CYP450 2D6 and CYP3A4.[21]

The sulfoxide on Prilosec (**11**) may be oxidized by S-MPH and CYP2D6 to provide the corresponding sulfone **22**, which loses its biological activity. The sulfoxide may be reduced as well into its corresponding sulfide, which losses its biological activity as well.

As far as the benzimidazole ring is concerned, aromatic hydroxylation at C-6 (see Fig. 10.2) is the prominent metabolic pathway in dogs. This is a great example where Mother Nature does C–H activation with stunning ease and precision! We organic chemists have a long way to go to mimic what enzymes (e.g., CYP450) can do. Also on the benzimidazole ring, the O-demethylation of the 5-methoxyl group is accomplished by S-MPH and CYP2D6 to afford 5-O-desmethyl-omeprazole (**21**).

The major metabolic pathways are summarized in Fig. 10.2.[21]

Now is an opportune time to address the question: Are Prilosec (**11**) and Nexium (**1**) the same *in vivo*? The answer is more nuanced than a simple "yes" or "no."

On one hand, it is likely that Nexium (**1**) is converted to the (*R*)-diastereomer **1′** via the intermediacy of benzimidazoline **15** (Fig. 10.3).

However, the metabolism rates for Nexium (**1**) and (*R*)-diastereomer **1′** are *not* the same. This should not be surprising because the enzyme that catalyzes the metabolism, CYP450, is chiral. Therefore, chiral compounds, even enantiomers *could* be metabolized differently and in particular case, the two enantiomers *are* metabolized differently. AstraZeneca (Hässle later became a part of AstraZeneca after a series of mergers) demonstrated a difference of pharmacokinetics between Nexium (**1**) and *R*-diastereomer **1′** *in vitro* and *in vivo*.[26]

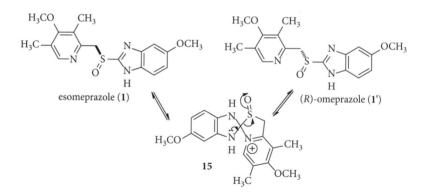

Fig. 10.3. Proposed possible *in vivo* isomerization of the (S)-isomer **1** to the (R)-isomer **1′**

For in vitro investigations, AstraZeneca incubated the two enantiomers with human liver microsomes; the results are summarized in Fig. 10.4.[26] One immediately notices that CYP2C19 plays the most important role for in vitro metabolism, whereas CYP3A4 and CYP2D6 are the major forces for the metabolism in vivo (see Fig. 10.1). For Nexium (**1**), CYP2C19 is responsible to oxidize 27% of **1** to 5-hydroxyl esomeprazole and 46% to 5-O-desmethyl esomeprazole. So CYP2C19 is responsible for metabolizing 73% of the API. The remaining 27% of **1** is metabolized by CYP3A4 to its corresponding sulfone **22**, which is not an active metabolite.

On the other hand, CYP2C19 metabolizes nearly all of R-diastereomer **1′** to the tune of a whopping 98%, of which 94% is 5-hydroxyl R-omeprazole.

While Fig. 10.4 depicts the different *ratios* of metabolites from Nexium (**1**) and R-enantiomer **1′** in vitro, the figure does not reflect the rates at which the two compounds are metabolized. CYP2C19 obviously is the most important isoform of the CYP450 enzymes and it metabolizes Nexium (**1**) at a *slower rate* than that for the R-enantiomer **1′**. For instance, Nexium (**1**) is converted to 5-hydroxyl esomeprazole ten time slower than the R-enantiomer **1′**.

As a consequence, it is not only the metabolite distributions that are different for **1** and **1′**; the R-enantiomer **1′** is cleared faster than **1**, as reflected by their in-

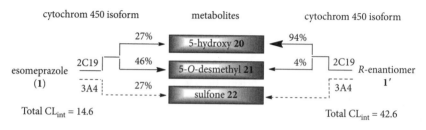

Fig. 10.4. In vitro Metabolism of Esomeprazole (**1**) and the R-Enantiomer **1′** in Human Liver Microsomes.[26] Adapted with Permission

trinsic clearance values (CL_{int}) as 42.6 and 14.6, respectively.[26] Because the CL_{int} values are 3-fold higher for the R-enantiomer **1'**, the end result is that the concentration time curve (AUC) is higher for Nexium (**1**) than that of (R)-omeprazole **1'**.

In conclusion, Nexium (**1**) is *more* bioavailable *in vitro* than its corresponding (R)-enantiomer **1'**. By extension, Nexium (**1**) is *more* bioavailable than Prilosec (**11**), a fact that has been confirmed experimentally. In vivo pharmacokinetics also demonstrated that Nexium (**1**) is *more* bioavailable than its corresponding (R)-enantiomer **1'**.[26]

Decades of clinical use solidly demonstrated favorable benefit/risk profiles for all PPIs including Nexium (**1**) and Prilosec (**11**), as well as Prevacid (**12**), Protonix (**13**), and Aciphex (**14**). The most frequent (in a relative term) side effect for PPIs are bone fractures involving the hip, wrist, forearm, and other weak sites. However, the bone fracture incident rate for people taking PPIs is only slightly higher than the control group within the same age population. In all, PPIs have only 1–5% incidents of minor adverse drug reactions.[27] This is on par with histamine-2 receptor antagonists such as cimetidine (Tagamet, **2**), ranitidine (Zantac, **3**), famotidine (Pepcid, **4**), and nizatidine (Axid, **5**).

The other known possible side effects that have been associated with PPIs are cardiac arrhythmias, and *Clostridium difficile* infections.

However, since Nexium (**1**) is metabolized by CYP2C19 and CYP3A4, it is prone to have potential DDIs with drugs that use the same CYP450 isoforms for their metabolism. For instance, the anti-platelet drug clopidogrel (Plavix, see chapter 2) is metabolized by CYP2C19, among other isoforms of CYP450. Taking clopidogrel together with PPI has been reported to increase both the anti-aggregation effects (good) and the risk of cardiovascular ischemic events (bad).[28] Because there is a certain amount of CYP2C19 busily engaged in metabolizing PPIs, clopidogrel's bioavailability subsequently is boosted.

Unique to PPIs though, is that they inhibit the secretion of gastric acid, which helps drugs dissolve in the stomach. Therefore, taking Nexium (**1**) may reduce the bioavailabilities of other concurrent medications ranging from 10% (phenytoin) to 50% (e.g., ketoconazole, atazanavir).[28]

It is fair to ask the question: "Do enantiomers and racemic mixtures have the same safety profile?"

Again, it depends on the drug. The most tragic example is thalidomide. While (R)-thalidomide was effective against nausea, (S)-thalidomide was highly teratogenic in humans!

The occurrence of hematological effects was known to be different for Nexium (**1**), and omeprazole (**10**).[29] In 2012, a meta-analysis of the French Pharmaco-Vigilance Database (FPVDB) indicated that Nexium (**1**) induces more hematological disorders than Prilosec (**11**).[30] The difference is possible the result of different metabolite (**20**, **21**, and **22**) distributions between Nexium (**1**) and Prilosec (**11**).

■ 3 SYNTHESIS

3.1 Discovery Route

3.1.1 Synthesis of Prilosec[31–35]

The synthesis of Prilosec (11) provides a good foundation for the synthesis of Nexium (1).[31–33]

As shown in Scheme 2, the synthesis began with 3,5-dimethylpyridine (23). Addition of methyllithium onto the pyridine ring of 23 resulted in 2,3,5-trimethyl-pyridine (24). Oxidation of 24 with hydrogen peroxide then provided the pyridine N-oxide 25. Nitration of 25 using the traditional conditions with a nitronium ion generated from mixing HNO_3 with H_2SO_4 gave rise to nitro-pyridine 26. An S_NAr then took place between 26 and methoxide in methanol to install the desired methoxy group on 27, with the nitro group on 26 as the leaving group. A subsequent Boekelheide reaction on N-oxide 27 led to hydroxymethyl-pyridine 28, which was converted to pyridylmethyl chloride 29 by direct chlorination of alcohol 28 using thionyl chloride.

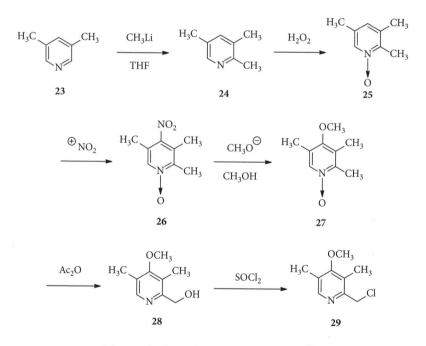

Scheme 2. Synthesis of pyridylmethyl chloride 29[31]

With the pyridine fragment prepared in the form of chloride 29, the synthesis of omeprazole (10) is made more straightforward by building the benzimidazole ring. As shown in Scheme 3, methoxyphenylene diamine (30) was treated with potassium ethylxanthate to afford benzimidazole-thiol 31. The coupling of thiol 31 and chloromethyl-pyridine **29** was then facilitated by treatment with NaOH in refluxing EtOH/H$_2$O. Subsequently, the oxidation of the resulting sulfide **32** (pymetazole) was easily carried out using *m*-CPBA in CHCl$_3$ to deliver omeprazole (**10**). An improved transformation of pymetazole (**32**) to omeprazole (**10**) was patented in 1991.[34] The invention involved carrying out the *m*-CPBA oxidation of pymetazole (**32**) in CH$_2$Cl$_2$ at a substantially higher pH of 8.0 to 8.6 using KHCO$_3$ as the buffer. The reaction mixture was subsequently extracted with aqueous NaOH. The separated aqueous phase was then treated with an alkyl formate (e.g., methylformate), maintaining the pH > 9, allowing omeprazole (**10**) to crystallize. Another improved sulfide oxidation was patented in 2000 employing EtOAc as the solvent for the last step.[35]

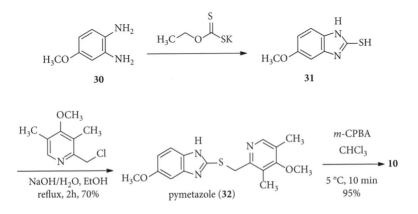

Scheme 3. Synthesis of Omeprazole (**10**)[33]

3.1.2 Synthesis of Nexium

A small amount of Nexium (**1**) in the early discovery phase was conveniently accomplished via an HPLC separation of the two enantiomers of Prilosec (**10**).[36] Somewhat larger-scale separations (also in discovery phase) was achieved by a reverse phase HPLC of the two diastereomers of an alkylated omeprazole.[37,38] In order to install the requisite chiral auxiliary, a "handle" was required for tethering. This was installed by treating **10** with formaldehyde followed by chlorination with thionyl chloride to afford chloromethyl-benzimidazole **33**. Here the alkyl group also serves as a linker to a chiral auxiliary. Subsequently, treatment of **33** with (*R*)-(–)-mandelic acid (**34**) in the presence of NaOH under phase transfer catalysis (PTC) conditions gave ester **35** as a mixture of two diastereomers. The pair of diastereomers was then separated by reverse phase HPLC to render the pure diastereomer **35a**. Removal of the (*R*)-(–)-mandelic acid chiral auxiliary was achieved by a brief exposure of ester **35a** to a NaOH solution. Finally, magnesium salt formation using MgCl$_2$ then delivered Nexium (**1**).

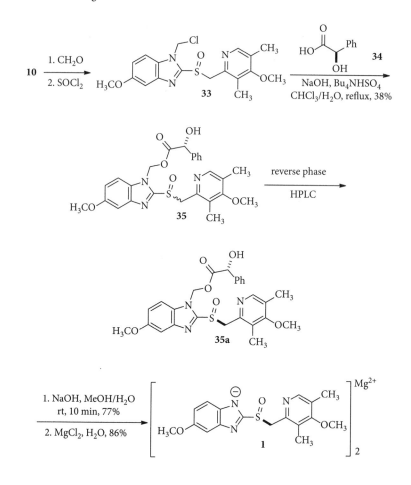

3.2 Process Route

3.2.1 Asymmetric Oxidation of the Sulfide

The advent of asymmetric synthesis methodology has had a tremendous impact on both academia and industry. For example, the Sharpless epoxidation has become a staple in the construction of chiral building blocks. Asymmetric oxidation of sulfides (also known as the Kagan oxidation) has been explored and applied in process synthesis and manufacturing to make chiral sulfoxides.

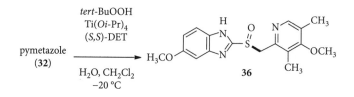

The initial direct application of the Kagan conditions to the prochiral sulfide on pymetazole (**32**) gave little stereoselectivity with only a meager 5% *ee*. Unexpectedly, simple addition of the Hünig base boosted the *ee* of **36** to 60% without any additional changes of the reaction conditions.[39] This incident exemplifies the important contributions that process chemists can make to large-scale preparations of APIs.

Further fine-tuning of the reaction conditions revealed that using toluene instead of CH_2Cl_2 and slightly elevated temperature at 30 °C offered **36** in >90% yield with 90% *ee*. At the end,[40–43] asymmetric oxidation of pymetazole (**32**) was accomplished by employing cumene peroxide, Ti(Oi-Pr)$_4$, Hünig base, and a *catalytic* amount of chiral ligand D-(−)-diethyl tartrate to fashion sulfoxide **36** in >98% *ee*. Conversion of **36** to the corresponding magnesium salt **1** was then easily accomplished by treatment with Mg(OMe)$_2$. The asymmetric oxidation approach has been used for both the large-scale and manufacturing processes.

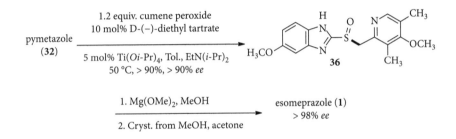

3.2.2 Biooxidation

Biotransformations have become recognized as a viable method for chemical transformations due to their environmentally friendly conditions. In this particular case, oxidation of the sulfide **32** can be carried out via biooxidation.[44,45] The screening process gave enantiomerically enriched **36** with *ee* of 56–99%. In particular, *Penicillium frequentans* BPFC 386, *P. frequentans* BPFC 585, and *Brevibacterium paraffinophagus* ATCC 21494 all resulted in >99% *ee*.

$$\text{pymetazole (32)} \xrightarrow[\text{BPFC 386}]{\textit{Penicillium frequentans}} \textbf{36}$$

Similarly, sulfides **37** and **38** were biooxidized to the corresponding enantiomerically enriched sulfoxides, (−)-lansoprazole (**12′**) and (−)-pantoprazole (**13′**). These biotransformation processes are still at the exploratory stage. The concentration of the substrate is generally minute—in the ppm range. As a result, this method is not suitable for large-scale processes.

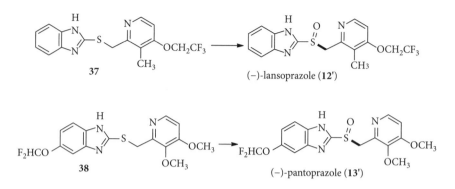

37 → (−)-lansoprazole (**12'**)

38 → (−)-pantoprazole (**13'**)

■ 4 CONCLUDING REMARKS

After the tremendous success of H_2 histamine receptor antagonists and proton pump inhibitors, it is now understood that ulcers are caused by a bacterium.

Warren and Marshall at the Royal Perth Hospital in Western Australia discovered *H. pylori* in 1982 with the aid of a flexible fibroptic gastroscope. They succeeded in isolating and growing the bacterium in vitro. Marshall even used himself as a guinea pig to test the bacterium by drinking a solution containing *H. pylori* and promptly developing an ulcer.[1,46] After that experiment was published, the causation of gastric inflammation by *H. pylori* was indisputably established.[1] Warren and Marshall were awarded the Nobel Prize for Physiology or Medicine in 2005 for their discovery of the bacterium *H. pylori* and its role in gastritis and peptic ulcer disease.

As a consequence of Warren and Marshall's discovery, a reasonable treatment of ulcer should be a combination of an antimicrobial to eradicate the bacterium and another drug such as a H_2 histamine blocker or a PPI.

■ 5 REFERENCES

1. *Helicobacter pylori, Gastritis and Peptic Ulcer,* Malfertheine, P.; Ditschuneit, H., Eds.; Springer: Heidelberg, Germany, 1990.

2. Konturek, S. J. *J. Physiol. Pharmacol.* **2003**, *54*, S3, 43–68.

3. Popielski, L. *Pfluegs Arch. Ges. Physiol.* **1920**, *178*, 237–259.

4. Parson, M. E.; Ganellin, C. R. *Br. J. Pharmacol.* **2006**, *147*, S127–S135.

5. Ganellin, C. R. Cimetidine, in *Chronicles of Drug Discovery: Volume 1 (ACS Professional Reference Books),* Bindra, J. S.; Lednicer, D., Eds.; Wiley: New York, 1983, pp. 1–38.

6. Ganellin, C. R. Discovery of Cimetidine, Ranitidine and other H_2 receptor histamine antagonists, in *Medicinal Chemistry: The Role of Organic Chemistry in Drug Research* Ganellin, C. R.; Roberts, S. M., Eds., Academic Press: London, 1994, pp. 228–254.

7. Ganellin, C. R. Development of anti-ulcer H_2 receptor histamine antagonists, in *Analogue-Based Drug Discovery,* Fischer, J.; Ganellin, C. R., Eds., Wiley-VCH: Weinheim, Germany, 2006, pp. 71–80.

8. Sjöstrand, S. E.; Olbe, L.; Fellenius, E. The discovery and development of the proton pump inhibitors, in *Proton Pump Inhibitors (Milestones in Drug Therapy)*, Olbe, L. Ed.; Birkhäuser Verlag: Basel; 1999, pp. 3–20.

9. Olbe, L.; Carlsson, E.; Lindberg, P. *Nat. Rev. Drug Discov.* **2003**, *2*, 132–139.

10. Modlin, I. M.; Sachs, G. *The Logic of Omeprazole: Treatment by Design*, CoMed Communications: Philadelphia, PA, 2000.

11. Chieli, E.; Malvaldi, G. *Biochem. Pharmacol.* **1985**, *34*, 395–396.

12. Lindberg, P.; Brändström, A.; Wallmark, B.; Mattsson, H.; Rikner, L.; Hoffmann, K. J. *Med. Res. Rev.* **1990**, *10*, 1–54.

13. Lindberg, P.; Carlsson, E. Esomeprazole in the framework of proton-pump inhibitor development, in *Analogue-Based Drug Discovery*, Fischer, J.; Ganellin, C. R., Eds.; Wiley-VCH: Weinheim, Germany, 2006, pp. 81–113.

14. Berkowitz, B. A.; Sachs, G. *Molec. Interven.* **2002**, *2*, 6–11.

15. Carlsson, E.; Lindberg, P.; von Unge, S. *Chem. Brit.* **2002**, *38*, 42–45.

16. Rabon, E.; Chang, H. H.; Saccomani, G.; Sachs, G. *Acta Physiol. Scand.*, *Suppl. (Proc. Symp. Gastric Ion Transp., 1977)*, **1978**, 409–426.

17. Modlin, I. M. J. *Clin. Gastroenterol.* **2006**, *40*, 867–869.

18. Lindberg, P.; Nordberg, P.; Alminger, T.; Brändström, A.; Wallmark, B. J. *Med. Chem.* **1986**, *29*, 1329–1340.

19. Shin, J. M.; Sachs, G. *Dig. Dis. Sci.* **2006**, *51*, 823–833.

20. Lindberg, P.; Brändström, A.; Wallmark, B. *TIPS* **1987**, *8*, 399–402.

21. Regårdh, C. G.; *Scan. J. Gastroenterol.* **1986**, *118(Suppl)*, 99–104.

22. Renberg, L.; Simonson, R.; Hoffmann, K-J. *Drug Metab. Dispos.* **1989**, *17*, 69–76.

23. Hoffmann, K-J.; Renberg, L.; Olovson, S.-G. *Drug Metab. Dispos.* **1986**, *14*, 336–340.

24. Hoffmann, K-J. *Drug Metab. Dispos.* **1986**, *14*, 341–348.

25. Andersson, T.; Miners, J. O.; Veronese, M. E.; Tassaneeyakul, W.; Meyer, U. A.; Birkett, D. J. *Br. J. Clin. Pharmac.* **1993**, *36*, 521–530.

26. Andersson, T.; Hassan-Alin, M.; Hasselgren, G.; Röhss, K.; Weidolf, L. *Clin. Pharmacokinet.* **2001**, *40*, 411–426.

27. McCarthy, D. M. *Curr. Opin. Gastroenterol.* **2010**, *26*, 624–631.

28. Ogawa, R.; Echizen, H. *Clin. Pharmacokinet.* **2010**, *49*, 509–533.

29. Moachon, L.; Benm'rad, M.; Pierre, M.; Grimaldi, D.; Blanche, P. *Fundam. Clin. Pharmacol.* **2010**, *24(Suppl. 1)*, 83.

30. Bagheri, H. *Br. J. Clin. Pharmac.* **2012**, *36*, 886–889.

31. Junggren, U. K.; Sjöstrand, S. E. EP 0005129 (1979).

32. Kohl, B.; Sturn, E.; Senn-Bilfinger, J.; et al. J. *Med. Chem.* **1992**, *35*, 1049–1053.

33. Winterfeld, K.; Flick, K. *Arch. Pharm.* **1956**, *26*, 448–452.

34. Brändströn, A. E. WO 9118895 (1991).

35. Hafner, M.; Jereb, D. WO 0002876 (2000).

36. Erlandsson, P.; Isaksson, R.; Lorentzon, P.; Lindberg, P. J. *Chromatogr.* **1990**, *532*, 305–319.

37. WO 9208716 (1992).

38. Lindberg, P. L.; Von Unge, S. WO 9427988 (1994).

39. Lindberg, P. L.; Von Unge, S. US 5714504 (1998).

40. Pitchen, P.; Dunach, E.; Deshmukh, M. D.; Kagan, H. B. J. *Am. Chem. Soc.* **1984**, *106*, 8188–8193.

41. Cotton, H.; Kroström, A.; Mattson, A.; Möller, E. WO 9854171 (1998).

42. Holte, R.; Lindberg, P.; Reeve, C.; Taylor, S. WO 9617076 (1996).

43. Federsel, H.-J. *Chirality* **2003**, *15(Suppl)*, S128–S142.

44. Cotton, H.; Elebring, T.; Larsson, M.; Li, L.; Sörensen, H.; von Unge, S. *Tetrahedron: Asymmetry* **2000**, *11*, 3819–3825. Sulfide **32** was incubated with a variety of microorganisms in 50 mM Na_2HPO_4 buffer, pH 7.6 with 5–10 g/L dry cell weight and a substrate concentration of 1 g/L. The cells were incubated with the sulfide **32** on a rotary shaker at 28 °C for 18–20 h.

45. Holte, R.; Lindberg, P.; Reeve, C.; Taylor, S. WO 9617076 (1996).

46. Meyers, Morton A. *Happy Accidents, Serendipity in Modern Medical Breakthroughs,* Arcade Publishing: New York, 2007, pp. 99–113.

■ INDEX